Group B Strep Explained

Sara Wickham

AiMS

There for your mother
Here for you
Help us to be there for your daughters

© AIMS 2014

Published by AIMS

www.aims.org.uk

Association for Improvements in the Maternity Services

Registered Charity number 1157845

ISBN: 978-1-874413-37-0

Cover Image: Pipa Derrick

Printed in the Czech Republic by Printo

Typeset by Triarchy Press, Axminster, UK.

Acknowledgements

I never tire of beginning these books by thanking all of the women who work so hard and so freely for AIMS with the goal of improving maternity care; I am in awe of the passion that you all have and it is always a pleasure to work with you.

Several AIMS committee members and other people were particularly involved in making this book. Virginia Hatton midwifed this project brilliantly from conception to birth and both she and Nadine Edwards have provided amazing and ongoing support in numerous dimensions. Shane Ridley deserves a special thank you for helping the book move from first draft to final publication, while Beverley Beech, Debbie Chippington Derrick, Gina Lowdon, Chloe Bayfield, Pipa Derrick, Ceri Durham, Vicki Williams and Emma Ashworth have provided support and ideas, read and commented on pages and pages of work, supported numerous elements of the design and production process, worked on related projects and been equally valiant, knowledgeable and kind in a huge variety of ways: thank you all.

I also want to thank all of the women who sent me their stories – I hope I have honoured all of your different viewpoints – and the people who responded to my requests for information on my website and via social media. Thanks to midwives and obstetricians Vicky Carne, Katy Coles White, Lyn Crocker-Eakins, Ffion Dalziel, Lorna Davies, Julie Frohlich, Sharon McKenna, Kirsten Small and Suyai Steinhauer, all of whom helped me check facts or access information that I needed in different ways. Of all the people previously mentioned I want to say a special thank you to Kirsten for reading and commenting on the entire book, to Debbie for checking my maths and to my favourite microbiologist, who didn't want to be named in case I wrote anything too controversial! Any mistakes or misunderstandings are all mine. Finally, and by no means least, I want to thank my partner Chris, who sat through three months' worth of conversation about bacteria and made most of the cups of tea that fuelled the writing of this book.

About AIMS

The Association for Improvements in the Maternity Services (AIMS) has been at the forefront of the childbirth movement since 1960, run entirely by unpaid volunteers. AIMS is a voluntary organisation established in 1960 and became a Registered Charity in 2014.

AIMS' day-to-day work includes providing independent support and information about maternity choices and raising awareness of current research on childbirth and related issues. AIMS actively supports parents and healthcare professionals who recognise that, for the majority of women, birth is a normal rather than a medical event. AIMS campaigns tirelessly on many issues covered by the Human Rights legislation.

Contents

Author's Foreword

As I begin this book, I am all too aware that this is an incredibly emotive area for some people. In the weeks before I began to write, I invited friends, colleagues and contacts to send me their thoughts and comments on what they would like to see included. I have tried to make sure that I have addressed as many of the questions that I received as possible, even if sometimes the best I can do is to acknowledge the importance of the question and say that we do not know the answer.

The diversity of opinions reflected in the responses that I received did not really surprise me, for I have given many talks on this topic over the past few years and am used to hearing a range of views. But I still want to say a little bit about this before we begin the book proper because, if you are new to this area, I think it may be valuable for you to know that there are some very distinctive and different perspectives on this topic. Also, because I think it is vital for people to understand how information from different sources will be influenced by the experiences, beliefs and opinions of the people offering it, I would like to be very open and honest about how I have approached this book so that you can make your own judgment about the value of this (and hopefully all other) information to you.

Quite a lot of the information that is available online and from group B strep-related organisations is written by people who have either lost babies themselves because of group B strep (GBS), or who spend time supporting families who have gone through this. In fact, the authors of the most significant medical review of this area note that pressure from parents and the media was a factor in the introduction of guidelines for GBS prevention (Ohlsson and Shah, 2014). It is completely understandable that people who have had tragic experiences want to prevent others from experiencing similar things, but I think it is important to understand that decisions relating to this area are not cut-and-dried and that there are, as always, multiple dimensions to this picture.

I received a couple of emails from women who had lost babies to GBS disease asking if I would tell their stories in full in this book, because they felt that these stories would be more likely to make other women accept (or even demand) the tests and antibiotics that I discuss herein. But I received ten times as many requests from women asking me not to share such stories because they felt it was unfair to (in their words) *'play the dead baby card'* in order to try to persuade people to accept intervention in a situation where the issues are more complex and less clear than is sometimes portrayed. These women explained that they had felt bullied by people, professionals or organisations who were seeking to use emotion to persuade them to take a particular course of action.

You won't find these stories in this book, but that is as much because there isn't room as it is about my having made a conscious decision to exclude them. I have included women's words here and there to illustrate points, but overall I have tried to stick to a fair and reasoned discussion of the issues, because I don't think it's appropriate that I or anyone should try and persuade you to take a particular course of action. I cannot possibly know what it is to walk in your shoes, live in your body or grow your baby; we all have to make decisions based on our beliefs, experiences, faith, personal circumstances and/or family situation. Now that you know such stories exist, you can, should you want to, go and look for them – they are not difficult to find.

In our culture, you will encounter claims that childbirth is risky and arguments that medical intervention is essential far more often than you will hear the other side of the story. The gist of the other side of this story begins with the assertion that birth is generally a very safe and normal journey but that, no matter what we do, women and babies will sometimes encounter problems such as GBS disease. The questions that I am considering in this book are about whether and how we can and should try to predict and treat the problem of GBS disease. This is a tricky topic because the research evidence is confusing and sometimes lacking and the treatment currently used in an attempt to prevent GBS disease – intravenous antibiotics, given when a woman is in labour – carries risks, consequences and side effects. We don't have good evidence that this is an effective thing to do and the current approach means that lots of women end up having antibiotics which they do not need, and which may cause harm to them and/or their babies. Clearly, this is not ideal. Women who are found to have GBS in pregnancy are sometimes told they must give birth in hospital, even if they had planned to give birth at home or at a birth centre. Ironically, going to hospital also means they are then exposed to even more bacteria.

I don't want to only give you this side of the story either though. I want to try and be as balanced as I can, and give you information from a number of different perspectives so that you can make the decision that is right for you. But in order to do that, I felt I needed to begin by telling you that these different perspectives do exist, and that this book is not just about sharing 'facts' (if only such things existed!) but about unpacking the different perspectives a bit so that you can work out what you think and feel and figure out what that right decision is - for you, your baby and your family.

These perspectives go all the way back to the way we think and talk about bacteria, so that's where I am going to begin; with a brief overview of the relationships that we humans have with bacteria and the language that is used to talk about these tiny organisms and the way they affect our bodies and babies. Part one of the book introduces some of the background to this area and parts two and three look at screening and treatment, respectively. Part four looks at some of the wider issues, including what happens after the baby is born and provides easy-to-find answers to the questions that women asked me to address in the book. We are aware that the book contains some repetition. This is because the issues are complex, and repeating some of the key factors can help people make sense of them. Also, not all readers will read this book from cover to cover like a novel; some women will need to access information on one element of this quickly, or are only interested in one area, yet they still need background information.

You will find all the references and a page of resources at the back of the book but I sometimes write about recent research on this topic, so you might like to visit and put GBS into the search engine on my website (www.sarawickham.com) and see if there is anything else of interest to you there. AIMS also has lots of information on its website at www.aims.org.uk.

I hope this book serves you and your family well.

Sara Wickham. Wiltshire, England. Summer 2014.

Part One: Introducing the Issues

The issues surrounding GBS and GBS disease are complex, and there are some basic issues, terms and concepts that need to be explained before we can really get into discussing the current situation and the research evidence. This first part of the book introduces some of those key issues and concepts so that we can draw upon them in later sections.

A brief introduction to human-bacteria relationships

Bacteria are essential to the continuation of human life as we know it. These tiny organisms play a critical role in decomposition, in the making of cheese, yogurt and other fermented dairy products and in all manner of modern technological and industrial processes from the manufacture of drugs to the cleaning up of oil spills.

Human beings also have many bacteria living on and within our bodies. As far as the human body is concerned, individual types of bacteria may be helpful, harmful or benign. In some cases, the nature of a particular kind of bacteria (that is, whether it is helpful, harmful or benign) can change according to circumstances. We actually know very little about this area, which is a growing science, although what little we do know is fascinating, and we are beginning to realise that bacteria may be far more important to us than we have previously imagined.

For instance, we have within our bodies many helpful bacteria such as the well-known *Lactobacillus acidophilus* which is one of a number of bacteria that helps us to digest food. *Lactobacillus acidophilus* can also be used to make yogurt which can be used to treat vaginal infections as well as eaten for nourishment. Because both the bacteria and the human host benefit, the relationship between human beings and *Lactobacillus acidophilus* is described as mutualistic. Indeed, many people are aware that fungal infections such as thrush can become a problem when the bacteria that keep them in check are removed, for instance after someone takes antibiotics.

Well-known examples of bacteria that are usually harmful to the human body include *Salmonella enterica*, *Clostridium tetani,* which causes tetanus, and *Mycobacterium tuberculosis*. The relationship between human and bacteria in these examples is described as parasitic, because the bacteria gains at the expense of its human host. These bacteria are also often referred to as pathogens, and the simple definition of a pathogen is something that causes disease.

But sometimes bacteria live in (and thus benefit from) their human host without doing anything particularly helpful or harmful. Where this occurs, the relationship between them is described as commensal. In fact, most of the bacteria that live within our bodies are thought to be commensalistic, although many people question whether our assessment of this might change over time as we discover more about some of the bacteria with which we co-exist.

Streptococcus agalactiae, otherwise known as group B streptococcus or GBS, and occasionally referred to as beta strep or haemolytic strep, is considered to be a commensal bacterium. It lives in the gut and/ or vagina of around a fifth to a quarter of people in the UK (with more on those exact figures and how they vary in different areas on page 20-21) and, for most of the time, it minds its own business and neither helps nor harms us. It can occasionally cause a urine infection in women and, even more occasionally, it can be the source of an infection in the womb after a baby has been born, but both of these situations are relatively uncommon. Serious GBS disease in adults is rare and almost always occurs in people whose bodies are already compromised by another condition.

Because they can live in the vagina and the rectum (which is very close to the vagina) GBS bacteria can be passed to a baby during birth. It is normal and healthy for a baby to pick up its mother's bacteria during birth, and usually this does not cause a problem. Indeed, this is necessary and beneficial. But occasionally a baby will become sick as a result of picking up GBS bacteria during birth, and, in rare situations, the illness that ensues can be fatal.

Much of the information in this book is about the screening tests and interventions which are offered to pregnant women and women in labour in an attempt to prevent GBS disease in babies. The screening tests are intended to determine which babies might have a higher chance of picking up GBS during birth and the treatments are intended to kill the bacteria which might cause these babies a problem.

A note about language and terminology

One of the things that always comes through loud and clear when I talk to women about this area is that some people are upset by the language and terminology used by some professionals and some of those who campaign for change in relation to GBS screening and treatment. This is for two main reasons. Firstly, some of these people have a tendency to use jargon, often unnecessarily, and this can confuse and complicate decisions more than is necessary. So I am going to try to define and explain every scientific term when it is first used in this book and not to over-use them where a non-scientific term can be used instead. Even more importantly, some women report that they feel dirty as a result of the language (and possibly the approach) that is used when GBS is discussed. They don't like being told that they are infected with something, or having information presented in a way that suggests they are unclean.

Some of this probably stems from the way in which, for the past few decades, Western culture as a whole has focused more on the kinds of bacteria that cause disease rather than presenting bacteria as organisms which can also be helpful (or, as yogurt adverts like to suggest, even friendly) or just benign. This isn't necessarily something that health professionals can easily address, and I would like to hope that this might already be changing as there is now far more focus on the positive elements of bacteria as part of the human microbiome, which refers to the total of all of the microorganisms that live on and in our bodies - including, of course, happy yogurt bacteria (Turnbaugh, et al., 2007, Collado, et al., 2012).

I have already explained that GBS bacteria are, in the vast majority of cases, a benign resident of the human body. When someone has a certain kind of bacteria living on or in their body, even if the bacteria are benign, they are sometimes said to be colonised by that bacteria. But while the biological definition of colonisation simply means that a species has moved to a particular area of the body or planet, in other contexts the term colonised is used to refer to the takeover of a place by settlers. This might explain why some women feel uncomfortable with the word.

If the bacteria is (or becomes) harmful, then terms such as *infection* or *infected* tend to be used, and these might well be appropriate when we are talking about a baby who has already become ill, but some people and texts use this term to refer to anybody who has GBS bacteria. This can feel like even more of an invasion and it isn't necessarily appropriate language when talking about a woman who simply happens to be one of the people for whom GBS bacteria is a normal part of their microbiome.

These issues were discussed by MacDonald et al., (2010) in their analysis of texts and practices relating to GBS. They noted that GBS is often personified, or endowed with human characteristics, which *'gives the impression that GBS is an enemy and out to kill "vulnerable" babies'*. They also found that many of the books and papers that discuss GBS use *'war talk ... words and phrases that might otherwise be found in the context of war and battle'*.

> 'In the obstetric and paediatric literature, a woman has a *"colonization status"* and infection statistics are *"attack rates"* ... Further examples increase the idea that the bacteria acts intentionally and strategically: *"immediate or delayed invasion of host defences"* and *"the amniotic fluid is infected from the ascending vaginal route"* as if part of a tactical invasion.' (MacDonald, et al., 2010: 49).

I am not sure that the perfect answer to the problem of what language we use exists at this point in time. There is a need for balance, and I don't want to underplay the severity of GBS disease by not using terms such as infected or infection when they are appropriate (such as when talking about a baby who has GBS disease), but militaristic language and language that might make people feel dirty or invaded is clearly inappropriate, so I am going to try and use everyday language – like carry, carriage or carrier – whenever possible and only use terms like colonised when I really have to, for instance because I am quoting research findings and I have to use the language of the original text in order to share with you what the authors found or said.

How common is GBS carriage?

We have known for many years that the prevalence of GBS carriage varies strongly with geographical region (Whitney, et al., 2004), even in relatively small areas. A systematic review of studies carried out in the UK showed that 18.1% of women carry GBS, but that there was substantial variation in the proportion of GBS carriers in different areas of the UK (Colbourn and Gilbert, 2007). Barcaite et al. (2008) determined that the range of GBS carriage in Europe also varied, with regional carriage rates of 19.7-29.3% in Eastern Europe, 11-21% in Western Europe, 24.3-36% in Scandinavia, and 6.5-32% in Southern Europe. Since then, a number of researchers have published studies looking at the prevalence of GBS carriage in their hospitals or regions, and the variation in this becomes even more marked when we consider studies carried out in different areas of the world. These are just a few examples.

- 1.8% of women (about 1 in 55) were found to carry GBS in Maputo, Mozambique (de Steenwinkel, et al., 2008).

- 7.7% of women (about 1 in 13) in one area of Bangladesh were found to carry GBS (Chan, et al., 2013).

- 8.3% of women (about 1 in 12) were found to carry GBS in a study in Lithuania (Barcaite, et al., 2012).

- Two studies in Korea found that 8% (about 1 in 12) (Lee, et al., 2010) and 10% (1 in 10) (Hong, et al., 2010) of women carried GBS.

- 14% of women (about 1 in 7) who were between 34 and 37 weeks of gestation were found to be carrying GBS in a region of The Netherlands. (Tajik, et al., 2014).

- 17.7% of women (about 1 in 6) were found to carry GBS in three hospitals in Beirut, Lebanon (Seoud, et al., 2010).

- In a study in Emilia-Romagna, Italy, 18.1% of women (between 1 in 5 and 1 in 6) were found to carry GBS (Berardi A, 2011).

- 19.5% of women (about 1 in 5) booked at a hospital in Oklahoma City, USA, were found to be carrying GBS (Knudtson, et al., 2010).

- In one German University hospital, 21.1% of women (almost 1 in 5) were found to carry GBS (Kunze, et al., 2011).

- A study in New Zealand found 22% of women (between 1 in 4 and 1 in 5) to be carrying GBS (Grimwood, et al., 2002).

- 23% of pregnant women (about 1 in 4) were found to carry GBS at a hospital in Dar es Salaam, Tanzania (Joachim, et al., 2009).

- An Australian study found 23% of women (about 1 in 4) to be carrying GBS (Garland and Kelly , 1995).

- 60.3% of women (about 3 in 5) were found to be carrying GBS in three communities in Zimbabwe (Mavenyengwa, et al., 2010).

A few studies have considered whether there are factors that affect the likelihood that a person carries GBS. A study by Stapleton et al. (2005) suggested that ethnicity, BMI and occupation may play a part, with their results showing that black women, women with a higher than average BMI and health care workers had higher rates of GBS carriage than average. Researchers in Barcelona, Spain, found that women who experienced higher ambient temperatures and humidity had a higher chance of carrying GBS (Dadvand, et al., 2011). It is important to understand that these studies, while very interesting, were also relatively small, and some of these findings were quite marginal. Larger studies in different areas may well show different things.

There may be other factors that affect the likelihood that a person carries GBS. We don't know whether vaginal GBS carriage changes with sexual activity or factors such as condom use, or whether having candida (thrush) or another bacterial infection in the vagina has an effect on GBS. We don't know whether GBS has a role that we don't yet understand, or whether it doesn't really belong in the vagina and it only appears because something is out of balance with the person's microbiome. It might be affected by a woman's diet, or by the state of her immune system. There are many things we have yet to discover.

The bottom line is that there is no way of knowing whether you carry GBS unless you have a test to find out. The general consensus amongst medical professionals is that GBS is not necessarily something that people 'get' and then have forever. This is because it is quite possible for a person to test positive for GBS one week and negative the next, and vice versa. However, we don't know how much of this is because GBS bacteria 'come and go' or because the tests aren't as sensitive as they might be. This is quite an important consideration when we come to look at the timing of tests for women who choose to have these in part two.

So how do you know if you carry GBS?

The usual way of determining that a woman is carrying GBS bacteria is for a laboratory to analyse a swab of her vagina and rectum (back passage) or perianal area, which is the area around the anus. The rectum or perianal area is almost always swabbed as well as the vagina because studies have shown that taking a vaginal swab alone is not as effective at detecting GBS carriage. It is thought that bacteria can be present in the rectal or perianal area but absent from the vagina and yet still transfer to the baby at birth. Colbourn and Gilbert's (2007) review, for instance, found that 14% of women were found to be carrying GBS when vaginal swabs are used, but this rose to the 18.1% that I quoted above when swabs of their rectal area were tested as well. I haven't found any data on the rates of GBS disease in relation to where a positive test was obtained from, however. Research has shown that it is as effective to swab the perianal area as inside the anus, and less unpleasant for women, who may find it uncomfortable and embarrassing to have a swab inserted into their anus (Jamie, et al., 2004, Trappe, et al., 2011). GBS can also sometimes be detected when a urine sample is tested for bacteria, but urine testing on its own is not commonly used to test for GBS.

The GBS swab test shouldn't be painful, but the woman will need to undress and lie on her back with her legs apart, which some women find embarrassing and/or uncomfortable, especially in late pregnancy or labour. The swabs are like long cotton buds and, if the test is performed by a midwife or doctor, she or he will insert the swab just inside the vagina, gently rotate it and then withdraw it. Then the midwife or doctor will insert another swab into the anus, rotate it and remove it or touch the swab to the outside of the anus, rotate it and remove it.

Because of the risk of introducing harmful bacteria into the vagina, the vagina should always be swabbed before the rectum or perianal area. Instead of doing the test themselves, some midwives and doctors will ask the woman if she would prefer to take a swab to the bathroom and perform the test herself. Like inserting a tampon or menstrual cup, this can be done in one of a number of positions, according to personal preference. If you decide to undergo GBS testing but do not like the thought of someone else carrying it out, you may want to ask if you can do this yourself. The swab is then placed in a tube which is labelled and sent to a laboratory for analysis.

A similar test in which a swab is used to take a sample from the upper or lower vagina may sometimes be offered to women who have symptoms of vaginal infection, such as itching, discomfort or an unusual or smelly discharge. The swab can be tested for a number of other different kinds of bacteria as well as GBS. Although it is not considered to be a common cause of vaginal infection, GBS is sometimes picked up on such a test. This is why, as I will discuss later, women need to be aware of the implications of having a swab test. More information on the types, timing and funding of testing can be found in part two of this book. I should note, however, that this testing is not routinely recommended in the UK, because a different approach to determining risk is used.

Neonatal GBS disease

We have already established that GBS is a bacteria which some people carry – quite normally – in their bodies and that, while we don't think it offers any particular advantage to the carrier, it is usually not harmful or unhealthy. GBS can exist in the vagina or rectum (among other places) and therefore, when a woman who carries GBS becomes pregnant and gives birth, the GBS bacteria can sometimes be transferred to her baby during labour and birth. Most of the time this is not a problem and women with GBS in their vaginas give birth to babies every day who are healthy and well. When we collect swabs from the skin of babies, GBS bacteria is detected about half of the time.

Most babies who carry GBS bacteria are healthy and well. About half of these babies have picked up GBS during their birth, and about half haven't. Unfortunately, every now and then a baby who picks up the GBS bacteria during pregnancy or childbirth becomes very ill.

Group B strep disease in newly born babies is said to occur in two time frames.

1. **Early onset group B strep disease** is the one we are focusing on in this book. It occurs during the first seven days of life, although 90% of cases begin within the first 24 hours of life. It is more likely to occur in babies who are born prematurely, who are small, whose mothers' waters broke more than 12 hours before they gave birth or who have one or more of a number of other risk factors (Ohlsson and Shah, 2014, Yagupsky, et al., 1991). It is almost – but not quite – exclusively seen in babies born to women who already carry the GBS bacteria. The general belief is that this is because, at this early stage, there are not many other ways for a baby to pick up the bacteria, but when women have babies in hospital then the babies are often handled by health care workers who may carry GBS on their hands. This is not something that has been discussed a lot in the literature. In fact, Ohlsson and Shah (2014) propose that, in the few cases where babies have been born to women who had negative GBS test results, there may have been false negative results or other test-related errors. When micro-organisms such as bacteria are transmitted from a mother to a baby, the term vertical transmission may be used.

Early symptoms of early onset GBS disease in the baby include fever (a high temperature), feeding difficulties, making grunting noises, irritability, lethargy (being limp or hard to wake), breathing difficulties, unusual heart rate and/or a blue-ish tinge to the skin (which is less easy to spot in darker-skinned babies). Not all babies with GBS disease will have all of these symptoms, and many babies who have one or more of these symptoms don't have early onset GBS disease. A baby with early onset GBS disease may develop septicaemia (infection of the blood), pneumonia (inflammation of the lungs) and/or meningitis (inflammation of the brain and spinal cord). A baby who is thought to be affected by GBS disease will be commenced on treatment as soon as possible, with that treatment including antibiotics which are usually given intravenously.

2. **Late onset group B strep disease** occurs between seven days of age and up to three months of age. Factors that increase the chance of a baby developing late onset GBS disease include non-white race and preterm birth (Yagupsky, et al., 1991). Late onset GBS disease is not usually associated with pregnancy and the baby is likely to have picked up the GBS bacteria after birth. In contrast to the vertical transmission of early-onset GBS disease, late onset GBS disease is said to be spread by horizontal transmission (Morinis, et al., 2011). There is no suggestion that late onset GBS disease is preventable by any pregnancy or labour-related interventions, and so we will not be looking further at this in this book.

The incidence and outcomes of early-onset GBS disease vary according to time, place and perhaps the measures that are being taken to reduce them, but a good summary of the UK statistics is given in the Royal College of Obstetricians and Gynaecologists (RCOG) (2013) information leaflet:

> "One in every 2000 newborn babies in the UK and Ireland is diagnosed with GBS infection. Although the infection can make the baby very unwell, with prompt treatment the majority (7 out of 10 of diagnosed babies) recover fully. However, 2 in 10 babies with GBS infection will recover with some level of disability, and 1 in 10 infected babies will die. Overall, 1 in 17 000 newborn babies in the UK and Ireland die from the infection." (RCOG, 2013: 1).

I think it is very important to add here that the mortality (death) risk from GBS disease is very different in babies born at full term and babies who are born preterm. The US-based Centers for Disease Control and Prevention (CDC, 2010) showed that preterm babies are at greatest risk if they get GBS disease, and the mortality rate of babies who were born at 33 weeks gestation or earlier and who get GBS disease is 20-30% (so between 1 in 3 and 1 in 5). The survival rate increases with gestational age and babies born at full term (after 37 completed weeks of pregnancy) have a far lower risk of dying if they get GBS disease, at 2-3%, (or between 1 in 33 and 1 in 50). In other words, the mortality risk from GBS disease is ten times more in preterm babies than in babies born at full term (after 37 weeks of pregnancy).

Let's return to the RCOG data, which began with the statement that 1 in 2000 babies is diagnosed with GBS infection. As about 1 in 5 women carries GBS we can deduce that about 400 of the mothers of these babies carried the GBS bacteria, and that about 1 in 400 women who carry GBS bacteria will have a baby who develops GBS disease. If we again go back to the RCOG data this shows that 1 in 17000 babies will die, so we can again deduce that about 1 in 3400 babies born to women who carry GBS bacteria will die from the infection, while another 2 of those 3400 babies will recover but have some level of disability. Although the figures do vary a bit, around half of the babies born to women with GBS bacteria pick up the bacteria during birth, but 99.85% of babies (1997 in 2000) born to women who carry GBS will be unaffected by death or disability. The fact that GBS disease in newborn babies is rare is one of the reasons that countries such as the UK have avoided recommending screening all women for GBS, although I appreciate that such statistics may be meaningless to the families whose babies are or have been affected by GBS disease.

Summarising the dilemmas

These figures show that GBS disease is rare. Improved sanitation and living standards and advances in health care have reduced the risk of infectious disease dramatically but this has also changed the balance so that previously rare conditions that are harder to prevent are now seen as the biggest problems to solve. This is the case with GBS disease. Because of advances in the areas mentioned above, it is now the most common cause of infection in newborns born at full term (Vergnano, et al., 2010, Stoll et al., 2011). (The most common infection in preterm babies is caused by the E. coli bacteria). This is why the focus on GBS has increased in recent years, although as we will see in part two of this book, preterm babies are more at risk from GBS disease than full-term babies are.

The first guidelines on GBS disease were published in the US (AAP, 1992; ACOG, 1992) and the first UK guideline was published by the RCOG in 2003. But these guidelines and the versions that have followed them are very different from each other. The US, Australia and some other countries have taken a very different approach to determining who is deemed to be at risk from the approach taken in the UK. Part two of this book looks at the different approaches to determining who is at risk.

Part 2: Screening, testing and determining who is at risk

There has been a movement in health care over the past few decades towards trying to identify people who are at risk of having a certain problem or disease. If we know that a person is at risk of something, an attempt can be made to either prevent it, or treat it in the early stages before it becomes serious. Such is the basis for recommendations about breast self-examination, regular check-ups for people with diabetes and the questionnaires administered to people in hospital to determine who is at risk of getting bedsores. This second part of the book looks at the guidance and evidence that relate to whether and how we should try and determine which babies are at risk from GBS disease.

Explaining screening

Pregnant women are offered more screening tests than any other group of healthy people. Most of the things that midwives and doctors do during pregnancy are screening tests. We check women's blood pressure and urine and palpate women's abdomens to see if their uterus and baby are the 'right' size, the 'right' way up and in the 'right' position, and this is only in the first five minutes of the antenatal appointment. All of these are screening tests, and if one of these measurements is not within normal limits, we tend to recommend some kind of action as a result. Depending on whether the screening test is looking for an actual problem or a sign that someone is at risk of a problem, the recommended action might be actual treatment or some kind of preventative measure (which is also called prophylaxis). So when clinicians first decided they needed to address the problem of GBS disease, it was perhaps inevitable that the first step would be to search for a way to effectively screen for the problem, although of course this is only useful if we also have an effective form of prevention or treatment to offer to those babies who are deemed to be 'at risk'. I'll look at the question of treatment in part three.

Two very different approaches to screening emerged, and both of them remain quite crude. A good screening test will identify as many of the people who have a particular problem as possible, while not identifying too many people as being at risk if they don't have the problem. These elements are referred to as sensitivity and specificity. Both of the current approaches to screening for GBS disease are reasonably good (although not perfect) at picking up most of the people who are at risk (that is, they are quite sensitive) but both pick up very high numbers of people who are not at risk (so they are not very specific). Given that the consequence of being defined as 'at risk' is to be offered antibiotics in labour – which, if you decide to have them, means having a cannula in your arm and (usually) being in hospital, and having antibiotics that have their own associated risks – this is by no means an ideal situation.

The first of these screening approaches is to offer all pregnant women a GBS test as they approach labour, as currently happens in the US and many parts of Australia. This is sometimes called culture-based screening and intravenous antibiotics are offered during labour to all women with a positive test for GBS. This means that, in the areas where this type of screening is used, somewhere between a fifth to a quarter of all pregnant women are being offered intravenous antibiotics in labour in the hope of preventing GBS disease, which some people consider to be significant over treatment.

Other countries, such as the UK and New Zealand, take a different approach. Rather than routinely offering laboratory testing for GBS and then offering treatment to all of the 20-25% of women who are found to carry this, antibiotic treatment is offered to women who have certain risk factors which may increase the chance of their baby getting an infection and also to women who have signs of infection (which might include a raised temperature and/or pulse, womb tenderness and/or an unusual vaginal discharge) before or during labour. Some people refer to this as risk-based screening. This approach still means that a lot of women are offered antibiotics, but not quite as many as with culture-based screening.

The choice to recommend risk-based screening in the UK was a deliberate decision on the part of the RCOG, and is in line with the recommendations of the UK National Screening Committee (2008). The RCOG (2012) has clearly stated that it does not recommend routine bacteriological testing for GBS carriage in the antenatal period, and will not do so, 'until it is clear that antenatal screening for GBS carriage does more good than harm and that the benefits are cost-effective' (2012: 3).

Sometimes, in countries that use risk-based screening, a woman happens to be found to be carrying GBS via a test that was carried out for another reason. The most common examples of this situation are where a woman has a urine test for possible urine infection or a vaginal swab is taken because a woman went to the hospital in late pregnancy with a possible problem. Where this occurs, practitioners will generally offer her antibiotics when she goes into labour. Antibiotics will also usually be offered to a woman who has undertaken a private GBS test whose result is positive. Again, however, women are not *routinely* offered a GBS test in the UK because the overall approach focuses on identifying risk factors that will make the baby more susceptible to the effects of GBS if it is present rather than testing for GBS carriage. If a woman is found to carry GBS, practitioners will offer treatment accordingly.

Homer et al. (2014) recently carried out an analysis of the existing international guidelines which found that both culture-based and risk-based approaches to the prevention of early-onset GBS could be recommended as reasonable approaches. They concluded that the standard of the guidelines in most countries was high and that there was a lack of clear evidence showing that either one of the approaches was better than the other. Individual women and practitioners may agree or disagree with the approach offered in their region, as the differences very much relate to overall beliefs about birth, health and risk. Some women living in areas that use risk-based screening disagree with this approach and choose to have a GBS test privately, while other women are very happy that the UK has resisted adopting an approach that would lead to even more women being offered antibiotics in labour and further restrict some women from being able to make the decisions that are right for them. Some women who live in areas which offer a 'test and treat' approach choose instead to ask questions, and they may or may not go on to test and/or treat for GBS. Because early-onset GBS disease is rare and the risks of antibiotics are significant, some women choose not to have any testing in pregnancy that might detect GBS unless they feel this is truly necessary for a different problem. This is in order to avoid being urged to take antibiotics for GBS, and in some cases because of a concern that a positive result may restrict a woman's options.

Who is considered at risk in the UK?

In this section, I am going to look briefly at the RCOG (2012) UK guidelines, and then go into more detail below. On this subject, the RCOG (2012) is almost totally in agreement with the National Institute for Health and Care Excellence (NICE), who provide national guidance and advice with the aim of improving health and social care in the UK (NICE, 2008a, 2012). Guidelines in this area are continually being updated and vary by country and sometimes region, so you may want to check online for the most recent and geographically relevant guidelines to you. This is not hard to do – putting "group B strep guidelines" and your country or region into a search engine should get you what you need.

Routine Screening

In both the RCOG (2012) and NICE (2008a) guidance on antenatal care, routine screening for GBS is not recommended, but if a woman is found to be carrying GBS (for instance from a urine or vaginal/ perianal swab test carried out for another reason, such as investigation of a vaginal discharge), the guidelines state that she should be offered antibiotics in labour.

- However, antibiotic treatment in pregnancy is not recommended 'for GBS carriage alone'. In other words, if a pregnant woman has been found to have GBS but has no signs of infection and there is no other reason to consider antibiotics, then these should not be offered at that point just because she has GBS. She might be offered antibiotics in pregnancy for other reasons, but she will only be offered antibiotics for GBS carriage once she is in labour.

This means that women who wish to be screened for GBS (which is not routinely available on the NHS in the UK) and who use a reputable private testing company should not find it difficult to get antibiotics in labour if they are found to be GBS positive. Women who have concerns that they may have a vaginal or urinary tract infection will usually find that their midwife or doctor will recommend sending off a swab and/or a mid-stream sample of urine, and the tests that are carried out on this may detect the presence of GBS. Again, if they are found to be carrying GBS, the RCOG (2012) recommendation is that they should be offered antibiotics in labour.

However, women who do not wish to be tested and/or treated for GBS also need to be aware of this element of the guidance, because both AIMS and myself are aware of many cases where women have been tested for GBS without realising that this would be the case, for instance when they have given a mid-stream urine sample to be tested for urine infection or if they have had a vaginal swab to assess the cause of a vaginal discharge in pregnancy. In both cases, health professionals have not specifically mentioned that the laboratory may detect GBS and that this will have implications for the woman's care and decision-making, as I will discuss throughout the book.

Women deemed to be 'at greater risk'

There are a number of circumstances in which babies are considered to be at greater risk of developing early onset GBS disease and where their mothers will be offered different care and/or antibiotics in labour:

- Where women are 'at term' (that is, at least 37 weeks pregnant) and their waters break before they go into labour, the current recommendation is that they are offered a choice of immediate induction of labour or induction of labour after 24 hours. (Of course, they can also decide to wait longer, and this is discussed in AIMS' book Inducing Labour: making informed decisions (Wickham, 2014)). Antibiotics are not recommended unless there are other risk factors. However, if a woman in this situation is already known to carry GBS, the RCOG (2012) guidance recommends that she has immediate induction of her labour along with antibiotics rather than waiting.

- Even if they are not known to have GBS, the RCOG (2012) recommends that women who have a temperature (pyrexia) greater than 38°C in labour should be offered antibiotics, including an antibiotic recommended for prevention of early onset GBS disease.

- If a woman has previously had a baby with neonatal GBS disease, the RCOG (2012) recommends that she should be offered antibiotics in labour regardless of her GBS status and suggests that testing is unhelpful as antibiotics would be recommended even if these were negative for GBS. This situation is discussed further on page 56-58.

Women who should not be routinely offered antibiotics

However, the guidance is clear that, unless they are known to have GBS (in which case antibiotics will be recommended, as above) or other risk factors, the following groups of women should not routinely be offered antibiotics in labour for GBS:

- Women in established preterm labour whose waters have not broken.

- Women whose waters have broken preterm and who are not in labour.

- Women who were found to be carrying GBS in a previous pregnancy but whose babies had no problems.

Some women in these situations will find that they are offered antibiotics as a general protection against any infection; the RCOG (2012) document is emphasising that they do not recommend antibiotics in a specific attempt to protect the woman's baby from GBS disease in these situations.

Women having a caesarean section

For women having a caesarean: *'antibiotic prophylaxis specific for GBS is not required for women undergoing planned caesarean section in the absence of labour and with intact membranes'* (RCOG, 2012: 4). In one respect this is a bit of a moot point, because all women who have a caesarean section will be given antibiotics before the baby is born unless they specifically request otherwise. But the antibiotics will be given just before or during the operation, which will not allow for the four hour coverage that is deemed to be beneficial for the baby. Although the RCOG (2012) does not specifically discuss the thinking behind this part of the guideline, it may have a practical basis, as it would be difficult to be able to time antibiotics effectively in women having planned caesareans, which are often delayed or postponed. In addition, the babies of women having planned caesareans may also be deemed to be at low risk of developing early-onset GBS disease where they are being born at term and the membranes are intact.

Does the evidence support the guidelines?

The RCOG (2012) provides references and arguments to support its position in each of these situations, although some of these areas have been researched more thoroughly than others. Below, I look at the evidence offered by the RCOG in relation to each of these situations, but within a wider context as well, including reference to other evidence and debates where appropriate.

Routine screening

The RCOG (2012) notes that GBS screening is a controversial area, and provides a number of justifications for following the recommendation of the UK National Screening Committee that routine screening should not be adopted in the UK. One of the reasons that the UK has not adopted routine screening is because of studies like that conducted by Oddie and Embleton (2002). In their analysis of babies who developed GBS disease, 78% of those babies were identifiable through risk factors, such as being born preterm, being born after the waters had been broken for more than 18 hours or being born to a woman who had a raised temperature in labour. It is important not to forget the babies who were not identifiable through risk factors alone, but the Cochrane review (discussed in a number of other sections of this book) found that while antibiotic prophylaxis has *"reduced the incidence of EOGBS disease, it has not been shown to reduce all causes of mortality or GBS-related mortality"* (RCOG, 2012: 2). The RCOG (2012) also cites and expresses concerns about the disadvantages of antenatal screening and treatment for the mother and baby which *"include* anaphylaxis, *increased medicalisation of labour and the neonatal period, and possible infection with antibiotic-resistant organisms, particularly when broad-spectrum antibiotics such as amoxicillin are used for prophylaxis"* (RCOG 2012: 2).

Some people and organisations make the argument that countries such as the UK and New Zealand who use risk-based screening should be following the same practices as the US and Australia, claiming that these countries have had better success at dealing with GBS disease. But it is not that simple. The US and Australia have different rates of GBS carriage and neonatal GBS disease from the UK, and there are also some significant differences in midwifery and obstetric practice, which might account for the difference in rates that are cited. Women giving birth in the US and Australia will, on average, experience more medicalised maternity care, including more vaginal examinations and other interventions which may affect the number of babies who get GBS. A small study by Knudtson et al. (2010) suggested that vaginal examination doesn't make a huge difference to whether a woman tests positive for GBS, and if anything the likelihood of testing positive for GBS is reduced immediately afterwards, but this study had a number of limitations and only looked at the results of a GBS test immediately following the vaginal examination. In many areas of the US, women routinely have intravenous drips in labour and other interventions which may explain the differences (and which may arguably make additional intravenous drugs less of an additional intrusion in labour, although this will depend very much on the feelings of the individual woman), and the caesarean section rate is also higher. For all of these reasons, caution should be used when making comparisons between policies and outcomes in countries which have such different approaches to maternity care. The RCOG (2012) reached the same conclusion and considered that *"extrapolation of practice from the USA to the UK may … be inappropriate"* (RCOG 2012: 2).

Offering antibiotics if GBS is found coincidentally

It may seem curious to some readers that the RCOG (2012) guidance recommends against routine screening for GBS yet recommends that women who are found to have GBS coincidentally (e.g. on a swab or urine sample which is taken to check for infection more generally) are offered treatment for this once they are in labour.

The RCOG (2012) offers little evidence in support of this part of the guidance, but the statements it makes about risk are very telling. It is clearly concerned that, in these situations, women who are known to carry GBS are at greater risk of having a baby with GBS disease than a woman whose GBS status is unknown and, mathematically, this makes complete sense. But whether this additional risk justifies treatment (which is discussed in part three) is for the individual woman to decide. Unfortunately, we do not have enough evidence, as the RCOG acknowledges in its use of terminology: *"it is not possible to accurately quantify these increased risks"* and *"it is likely that the risk of neonatal disease is increased"* (RCOG 2012: 3).

In some ways, the stance that the RCOG (2012) takes here is understandable, especially in the context of our modern culture where doctors and midwives often fear that they may get into legal or professional trouble if they do not 'do as much as possible'. But this element of the guidance can be seen as problematic from both sides of the GBS screening and treatment debate. Those who advocate for offering routine laboratory testing for GBS might ask why, if the RCOG is so concerned to treat GBS when it is found coincidentally, does it not recommend testing everybody? Those who are concerned about the downsides of treating for GBS carriage (whether in general, or just in the absence of other risk factors) and who are pleased that the RCOG has avoided recommending routine screening are confused as to why the RCOG offers treatment for GBS carriage found incidentally when there isn't much evidence to support this. The answer is that, in maternity care, tradition, fear and/or peer pressure sometimes trump science.

Not offering GBS treatment in pregnancy

This element of the guidance is fairly uncontroversial. The RCOG (2012) states that antibiotic treatment in pregnancy is not recommended 'for GBS carriage alone'. This is for a number of reasons.

1. Antibiotics will be offered in labour anyway, so offering them in pregnancy as well would incur an extra dose.

2. Even if antibiotics were given in pregnancy, the GBS bacteria could return before labour.

3. The baby is not considered to be in any danger from GBS during pregnancy, as it is protected within the bag of membranes which contains amniotic fluid.

4. Offering antibiotics in pregnancy would further increase the problem of antibiotic overuse.

A number of recent papers have expressed concern about the percentage of pregnant women who receive antibiotics in pregnancy (Adriaenssens, et al., 2011, Broe, et al., 2014), and in my research on this area, I haven't encountered anyone who argues against this point.

If a woman has symptoms of infection in pregnancy, however, this is a different matter, and antibiotics will be offered to treat those symptoms. In this situation, if a woman had been found to have GBS and was treated in pregnancy because she had symptoms of an infection (such as a high temperature and/or pulse, or vaginal discharge), she would still be offered antibiotics in labour because of the possibility that the GBS could return.

Women who were found to be carrying GBS in a previous pregnancy

As previously mentioned, the RCOG (2012) guidelines state that previous GBS carriage alone (that is, in the absence of other risk factors) is not reason enough to warrant screening or antibiotic treatment in the current pregnancy. Its justification for this appears to be statistical. It has calculated that:

> "If GBS was detected in a previous pregnancy, the likelihood of
> carriage in a subsequent pregnancy is around 38%. This gives
> a risk estimate of neonatal EOGBS disease of approximately
> 0.9 cases/1000 births versus a background risk of 0.5
> cases/1000 births or 2.3 cases/1000 births in women with
> GBS detected in the current pregnancy." (RCOG, 2012: 3)

Although it does not specifically state this, the above paragraph implies that the writers of the RCOG (2012) guidelines believe this slight increase in risk is too small to warrant screening and/or treatment. Women who do not want screening and/or treatment for GBS despite having been found to carry GBS in a previous pregnancy have used this element of the guidance to form the basis for a discussion with their midwife or doctor. Women who are concerned that they want to do everything possible to minimise their baby's chances of having

GBS disease and are happy to take on the risks of antibiotic use have challenged this position and/or undertaken private testing.

Again, women who were found to be carrying GBS in a previous pregnancy may wish to know that the RCOG (2012) notes that current evidence does not support screening for GBS in these women either. This is important, because I am aware of a number of geographical regions in which this element of the RCOG (2012) guidance is frequently ignored. Women who have been told that they need to have screening and/or treatment, or who are told that their options for place of birth or type of care are limited because they were found to have GBS in a previous pregnancy may wish to discuss this with their midwife or doctor.

Women who are having a planned caesarean section

It has become the standard of care in the UK and many other countries to offer intravenous antibiotics to all women who are having a caesarean section, for the benefit of the woman. This is embedded in the NICE (2011) caesarean section guidance, which the RCOG (2012) cites in support of its position on this. The NICE (2011) guideline focuses mainly on the fact that giving women prophylactic antibiotics just before they begin the operation has been shown to reduce the risk of maternal infection more than giving prophylactic antibiotics during the operation (NICE, 2011). However, the timing of this has varied between different versions of the guideline, and there is little data about the safety of this for the baby. NICE (2011) also emphasises to caregivers the importance of giving antibiotics that reduce the risk of endometriosis (a condition where tissue from the womb grows outside the womb, causing pain), urinary tract infection and wound infection. The CAESAR study collaborative group (2010) found that, even with routine antibiotics, around 17 per cent of women who have a caesarean section get an infection. The most recent Cochrane review in this area concludes that:

> "Based on the best currently available evidence, cephalosporins and penicillins have similar efficacy at caesarean section when considering immediate postoperative infections. We have no data for outcomes on the baby, nor on late infections (up to 30 days) in the mother. Clinicians need to consider bacterial resistance and women's individual circumstances." (Alfirevic, et al., 2010: 1)

Local policies vary in regard to which antibiotic is given.

Women who are having a planned caesarean section and who want to have antibiotics that may also offer coverage for GBS may wish to discuss this with their midwife or doctor. Women will not be consulted separately about the antibiotic – consent for surgery will assume consent for an entire package of care and interventions that are associated with and part of this, including intravenous antibiotics.

A couple of specific situations are worth mentioning here, although they will not apply to everybody. Women who are having an unplanned caesarean section and who have spent at least some time in labour before their unplanned caesarean operation may have already been offered antibiotics for their baby if their baby was deemed to be at risk. In addition, the NICE (2011) guidance on antibiotics for caesarean section also applies to women who have a caesarean in labour that they did not expect to have, so they will also be offered antibiotics for their own benefit. As this is a complex area, where women know they carry GBS and are very keen to have a particular antibiotic, they may wish to discuss ahead of time what would happen if they needed an unplanned caesarean section in labour. This would also apply if a woman had an allergy or a previous reaction to a particular antibiotic.

Studies highlighting specific risk factors in or around the time of labour

I will return to looking at the specific situations in which women many find themselves in a moment, but as there are a couple of useful studies which relate to several of the next few topics, it seems sensible to discuss these in one place and then relate their findings to these specific situations.

The first of these studies was published in the British Medical Journal by Oddie and Embleton in 2002. This is a fairly well-known and often-cited study in the field, because its authors made the case for a risk-based approach to GBS screening rather than for testing every woman for GBS. The authors wanted to find out how common early-onset GBS disease was, and to see if they could identify any particular risk factors for this. They collected details of babies who developed early onset GBS disease in one particular area of Northern England, and compared these babies with carefully matched babies who did not have early onset GBS disease. In total, 36 babies developed early onset GBS disease out of a total of 62,786. This is 1 in 1744 babies, and this figure differs slightly from the 1 in 2000 figure quoted by the RCOG (2012) because the RCOG data amalgamates the rates from several different studies, in the hope of ironing out local variation and statistical anomalies which can occur when smaller studies are used.

Oddie and Embleton's (2002) findings included the following:

- Premature babies (those born before 37 completed weeks of pregnancy) comprised 38% of all cases of early-onset GBS disease, and 83% (5 out of 6) of the babies who died from

GBS disease had been born before 36 completed weeks of pregnancy.

- 68% of the babies with early-onset GBS disease were born to women whose waters had broken more than 18 hours before they were born.

- 19% of the babies with early-onset GBS disease were born to women who had a temperature in labour.

These findings support those of the NeonIN surveillance network (Vergnano, et al., 2011), which carried out research to look at the pattern of neonatal infection in twelve neonatal units in England over a two-year period from 2006-2008. While Vergnano et al. (2011) looked at all causes of infection, and not just GBS, they found that GBS was responsible for 58% of all infections. This is, as I mentioned near the beginning of this book, one reason why GBS receives so much attention. Vergnano et al. (2011) also discovered that the majority of all infections occurred in babies who were born before 37 completed weeks of pregnancy and/or who had low birthweight of less than 2500g, with 82% and 81% of babies being in each of these categories, respectively. Unfortunately, we do not have good ways of accurately predicting which babies will be born with low birthweight.

Oddie and Embleton (2002) claimed that, had the recommendations in place at the time (which are reasonably similar to the current RCOG (2012) recommendations) been applied, 78% of the mothers of the babies considered in their research would have been offered antibiotics in labour. This doesn't mean all the babies would have been saved, however, as I will discuss further in part three. Oddie and Embleton (2002) calculated that the application of such guidelines would mean that 16% of all women would have been offered antibiotics during labour.

A couple of years later, Heath et al. (2004) aimed to assess the national incidence of GBS disease in the UK and Ireland through multiple forms of reporting. A similar study is underway on babies born in the UK between 2014 and 2015 - see www.rcpch.ac.uk/bpsu/GBS. Such data is hard to collect accurately, because of local variation, but the researchers went to a lot of trouble to collect as many cases as possible. Again, they found that 37% of babies who developed early-onset GBS disease were born before 37 completed weeks of pregnancy, and 44% were born more than 18 hours after their mother's waters had broken. This study did not report on maternal temperature in labour.

It is important to note that none of this means that all or even the majority of women in these situations will have babies who develop GBS. In fact, very few women in these situations will have babies who become affected by GBS disease. It is simply that these studies have helped identify babies who are at greater risk. It is also important to remember that babies born to women who do not carry GBS are not likely to get GBS disease even if they are born prematurely or a long time after the waters have broken. All that population-level studies can do is to suggest factors that may indicate that a baby is at higher risk. Women and their families then need to decide what they think and feel about their own situation in the light of this data and other information. We will look at each of these situations (and others) in more depth over the next few sections.

Women whose waters break at term before labour

The studies just discussed are the main evidence for the RCOG's (2012) stance that women who are known to carry GBS and whose waters break at term (after 37 completed weeks of pregnancy) and before labour starts are offered antibiotics in labour and recommended to have immediate induction of labour. Other studies (e.g. Dillon, et al., 1987 and Garland, 1991) have also found this to be a risk factor, but as both of these were carried out in other countries, where practice is different, the RCOG have understandably focused on data generated within the UK context.

As above, 68% and 44% of the babies with early-onset GBS disease in Oddie and Embleton (2002) and Heath et al.'s (2004) studies were born to women whose waters had broken more than 18 hours before their babies were born. There is little doubt that this was a relevant factor in the development of those particular babies' GBS disease.

However, it would be helpful if we also knew how many babies were born completely healthily after their mothers' waters had broken more than 18 hours before they were born, because this would help us to put the figures into perspective and assess the magnitude of the risk from the perspective of the woman making the decision. Neither study tells us this, because both studies looked specifically at babies who had GBS disease, not at what percentage of babies in different situations developed GBS disease. Nor do the relevant RCOG (2012) or NICE (2008a) documents help us understand how they have arrived at their calculations of the risk in this area.

We could try and work this out for ourselves, but please understand that the following calculation is extremely rough and unscientific, as it is worked out on crude data and relies on a number of uncheckable assumptions. We know that the rate of prelabour rupture of membranes at term is around 8-10% (NICE 2008b). Given that 62,786 live births occurred in the period of Oddie and Embleton's (2002) study, we could guess that somewhere between 5022 (8%) and 6278 (10%) of the women in that area at that time experienced their waters breaking before labour. Some of those women will have been less than 37 weeks pregnant, but we have no way of knowing how many, which is one reason why this is unscientific. As above, 25 of the babies in that population developed GBS disease. So if we put these very rough figures together we can make a very rough guess that, all other factors excluded, a baby born to a woman whose waters break before labour has around a 0.4% (1 in 250) to 0.5% (1 in 200) chance of developing GBS disease.

We mustn't forget that this is all women, regardless of GBS status, and of the 5022-6278 (or so) women who are in our imaginary sample, only some of them will be carrying GBS. What about if a woman knows she is GBS positive? Well, if we assume that a woman has to be carrying GBS in order for her baby to pick up early-onset GBS disease and choose the 21% carrier figure found by Colbourne and Gilbert (2007) and used by the RCOG (2012), we are now talking about 25 babies born to (roughly) 1054 to 1318 women. This takes the risk of early onset GBS disease in a baby born to a woman who knows she carries GBS and whose waters broke before labour to somewhere between 2.4% (1 in 42) and 1.9% (1 in 53). Again, these figures are incredibly crude, and individual factors may increase or decrease the level of risk. The AIMS book *Inducing Labour: making informed decisions* (Wickham 2014) contains more information about what options women have when their waters break early, but this doesn't specifically consider the issue of GBS.

Women who have a raised temperature in labour

This is one area in which the RCOG (2012) and NICE (2012) guidance seems to differ slightly. Citing both the Oddie and Embleton (2002) and Heath et al. (2004) studies in support of the following statement, the RCOG (2012) guidance states that:

> "Women who are pyrexial [have a raised temperature] in
> labour should be offered broad-spectrum antibiotics including
> an antibiotic for prevention of neonatal EOGBS disease.
> Intrapartum pyrexia (>38°C) is associated with a risk of
> EOGBS disease of 5.3/1000 (versus a background risk of
> 0.5/1000). In view of this increased risk, IAP should be offered
> in the presence of maternal pyrexia." (RCOG, 2012: 5)

The NICE (2012) guideline development group (GDG) expresses itself a bit differently, however:

> "The GDG concluded that suspected or confirmed
> chorioamnionitis [an infection of the baby's membranes] and
> intrapartum fever (>38°C) are risk factors for early-onset
> neonatal infection but they are not indications for intrapartum
> antibiotic prophylaxis to prevent early-onset neonatal infection;
> the woman might receive antibiotic treatment for her own
> benefit, and this would be covered by obstetric practice"
> (NICE , 2012: 88)

The actual figure in the research by Oddie and Embleton (2012) was that 19% of the babies in their research who were diagnosed with early-onset GBS disease were born to women who had a temperature greater than 38°C in labour. Unlike in the previous example, however, I have not been able to find reliable enough data on the percentage of women who have a raised temperature in labour to even perform a crude and unscientific calculation which might help a woman decide what to do in this situation. There are data from the US (e.g. Dillon, et al. 1987) but these are three decades old and gathered in a very different context.

It is significant that two UK guidelines differ on this point and illustrates how this comes down to interpretation of the statistics, risks and wider issues. It may also be worth noting that, while a woman whose waters break before labour will be considered by many people to be experiencing a variation of the normal, a raised temperature is not usually normal or benign (except when it has an obvious environmental cause, e.g. it is a very hot day or the woman has been in water which is hotter than ideal) and most midwives and doctors would be concerned about this. A raised temperature usually indicates the presence of an infection, and because infection can spread more quickly than usual in pregnant and postnatal women and babies, concern is probably warranted. However, a raised temperature can also be caused by other things, such as the use of epidural anaesthesia. The decision to take antibiotics or not is clearly still up to the woman and needs to be made within the wider context of the situation and any other relevant factors. A woman who has an elevated temperature in labour may, of course, have an infection caused by something other than GBS bacteria.

Women who are in established preterm labour but whose waters have not broken

According to the RCOG (2012: 5) guidance:

> "Women presenting in established preterm labour with intact membranes with no other risk factors for GBS should not

routinely be offered IAP unless they are known to be colonised with GBS."F

The RCOG (2012) do acknowledge that the chance of early-onset GBS disease is higher in babies who are born early than in babies who are born at term (which was also the finding of several studies including those by Dillon, et al. 1987, Garland, et al. 1991, Yagupsky, 1991, Håkansson and Källén, 2006 and Valkenburg-van den Berg, et al., 2009), but it urges caution in this area. Firstly, it points out that around half of all women who present at hospital in what is thought to be preterm labour will not actually give birth to their babies preterm. In some cases, labour will stop naturally, while in other situations medical intervention may help delay labour.

But the RCOG has concerns even where women go on to be in established preterm labour. Giving antibiotics to all women in this situation would mean a large number of women and babies would be exposed to antibiotics and the RCOG (2012) further adds that:

> *"As the risk of EOGBS infection in this group of infants is still low, prompt management of early-onset sepsis, if it occurs, is preferable to IAP for large numbers of women."* (2012: 5)

Its caution is also based on the fact that:

> *"women presenting in uncomplicated spontaneous preterm labour with intact membranes are the same group of women as those recruited to the ORACLE trial where there was evidence of harm in terms of adverse neurodevelopmental outcome including cerebral palsy in their infants at 7 years of age in the absence of any demonstrable benefit in the short term"* (2012: 4)

In the ORACLE trial (Kenyon, et al., 2001a, Kenyon, et al., 2001b) the babies who had antibiotics were found to have a higher likelihood of adverse neurodevelopmental outcome, including cerebral palsy, and functional impairment at 7 years of age compared to the babies who didn't have antibiotics. One of the antibiotics that was used in this trial and which caused particular problems (Co-amoxiclav) is now no longer used as a result of this finding, but the RCOG remains concerned about the potential for adverse effects where women are in premature labour and recommend that antibiotics are not given unless there are clinical signs of infection. It states that *"there is no evidence from long-term follow-up studies that other antibiotics, including penicillin, are safe"* (RCOG, 2012: 4)

If women have been found to carry GBS, however, antibiotics are offered. As always, the final decision rests with the individual woman.

Some people have been concerned about whether carrying GBS can increase the chance of premature labour. This question was considered by Valkenburg-van den Berg et al. (2009) who undertook a systematic review. They found no association between maternal GBS carriage during pregnancy and preterm delivery.

Women who are in established preterm labour whose waters have broken

The RCOG (2012) also state that antibiotics are not necessary in this situation:

> *"There is currently no evidence to show that the subgroup of women in preterm labour with ruptured membranes have greater benefit from IAP. The difficulty in balancing risks and benefits of IAP for women in preterm labour could be resolved by a randomised controlled trial."* (RCOG 2012: 4)

The exception, again, is where a woman is known to be carrying GBS, because all women who are carrying GBS are offered antibiotics.

In both this and the last scenario, antibiotics are only one of the factors to be considered, and decisions are better made on an individual rather than a population basis. As infection is one cause of preterm labour, a proportion of women will be offered antibiotics for that reason. In practice, there is a low tolerance for other risk factors in this situation, so women may be offered antibiotics anyway. There may never be good population-level guidance on this because, as well as a lack of evidence, there are so many individual factors that may have a bearing on a woman's decision.

Women whose waters have broken preterm and who are not in labour

This is another situation where GBS is only one of the factors to be considered and other issues, such as how many weeks pregnant the woman is, will need to be taken into account in weighing the risks and benefits of different courses of action. If a woman has preterm prelabour rupture of membranes after 34 weeks, for instance, the NICE (2008b, 2013) guidelines recommend that the maternity team should discuss the following factors with her before a decision is made about whether to induce labour, using vaginal prostaglandin:

- risks to the woman (e.g. sepsis, possible need for caesarean section)

- risks to the baby (e.g. sepsis, problems relating to preterm birth)

- local availability of neonatal intensive care facilities

As far as GBS is concerned, the RCOG (2012) guidelines state that:

"Antibiotic prophylaxis for GBS is unnecessary for women with preterm rupture of membranes … Antibiotic administration specifically for GBS colonisation is not necessary prior to labour and should not be given 'just in case'. If these women are known to be colonised with GBS, IAP should be offered. Induction of labour should be considered if there is suspicion of chorioamnionitis [an infection of the membranes]." (RCOG 2012: 5)

Since those guidelines were written, several papers debating this issue have been published. These all relate to two studies which use the acronym PPROMEXIL, which stands for *Preterm Prolonged Rupture Of Membranes - Expectant Management versus Induction of Labor.* Both the PPROMEXIL and PPROMEXIL-2 studies looked at women whose waters broke prematurely and without her going into labour, and considered whether it was better to induce labour or wait. The main studies in this project did not focus on GBS, so this data is for all women whose waters broke early and before they went into labour. Both of these studies found that the overall rate of infection was low. In fact, it was lower than had been thought – 4.1% at most, which is about 1 in 25 of the babies who are in this unusual situation. Both studies also found that induction of labour didn't improve the overall outcome compared to expectant management; also known as watchful waiting.

But the studies have sparked some debate in relation to GBS, because a later analysis of the PPROMEXIL-2 data which looked just at the women who were known to carry GBS showed that the babies born to these women did seem to benefit from immediate induction. The researchers found that 15.2% of the babies born to women who carried GBS developed early-onset GBS disease when they had expectant management compared to 1.8% of the babies who were delivered immediately (van der Ham, et al., 2012a, van der Ham, et al., 2012b). The problem is that the women and babies in this trial were at a large number of different hospitals, and the trial didn't specify whether or not they should have antibiotics; instead, this decision was made individually, or according to local protocol. This is a confounding factor which may affect the reliability of the results. While (as I will discuss in part four) there is mixed data on whether antibiotics are effective, the fact that we don't know who had antibiotics and/or other treatments and interventions makes it very hard to interpret this data. In any case, we ideally need good-quality randomised controlled trials to see if treatments such as this are effective.

While I was writing this book, several researchers, including Tajik et al. (2014), Zilberman et al. (2014) and Gilbert (2014) were discussing issues relating to this area in the literature, but the data aren't clear enough to suggest that the RCOG (2012) guidance is out-of-date in this area. We also need to bear in mind that most women in the UK won't know whether they carry GBS anyway, and as we are seeing, this knowledge does not come without consequences. Ultimately, it is another situation where, unfortunately, we don't have good enough evidence.

Women who have previously had a baby with neonatal GBS disease

As already mentioned, both the RCOG (2012) and NICE (2012) guidelines recommend antibiotics in labour for a woman who has previously had a baby with GBS disease, even to the point where the RCOG (2012) see offering antenatal testing to these women to be pointless because antibiotics would be offered in labour anyway. They also state that *"the risk of GBS disease [in this situation] is unquantified but is probably significantly increased"* (RCOG, 2012: 5).

One of the main reasons for the concern in this area is illustrated by a report of the case of a woman who had two babies with GBS disease. The summary of this paper reads:

> *"At each of two consecutive deliveries a woman gave birth to a baby that developed early-onset group B streptococcal (GBS) septicaemia. A low titre of serum antibodies to the type of the infecting GBS and persistence of the organism in the mother were demonstrated. This case confirms that mothers of GBS infected infants are at high risk of their future babies being similarly infected."* (Carstensen, et al., 1988: 201)

Although both of this woman's babies survived GBS disease and went on to be healthy, this paper provided one of the first published discussions of the idea that some babies may be particularly susceptible to GBS disease because their mother has a low amount of GBS antibodies, as was the case with the woman whose story featured in this paper. Carstensen, et al. (1988) state that *"mothers of infants with GBS septicaemia usually have antibody concentrations within or below the lower quarter of the reference area"*.

We don't know whether this really is a high-risk situation or whether the woman whose story was shared in the paper mentioned above had simply been the unlucky person for whom 'lightning struck twice'. Studies such as that by Schrag, et al. (2013) which have looked at the babies who have early-onset GBS disease also identify the fact that women had a previous baby with GBS disease as a risk factor. However, although GBS disease in a previous baby is known to be a risk factor and the possibility that some women have a low level of antibodies is a concern, no-one has actually managed to quantify the level of this risk (RCOG, 2012).

It is hard to understand why more work hasn't been done to try and better understand this situation, especially as this might be a big clue as to why GBS disease only affects a few babies. This seems to be a missed opportunity to find a way of identifying specific women whose babies may be at greater risk. Instead, work is underway to try and develop a vaccine to GBS, although it is uncertain how many women would want to have this given that the overall risk of GBS disease is low.

It is likely (though not, of course, inevitable) that women who have previously had a baby with GBS disease may already have a strong view on this, which is unlikely to be swayed by evidence. Some women in this situation are very pro antibiotics and pro campaigning, and others have had poor experiences with professionals and/or consumer campaigning groups during their prior experience and would prefer to avoid intervention as much as possible in future pregnancies. This is a very personal decision.

Other possible risk factors

The Cochrane review in this area lists other risk factors that have found to be correlated with an increased chance of a baby getting early-onset GBS disease. The RCOG (2012) has not considered these in its guidance, and although it does not provide an explanation for this, it is not hard to imagine why from even a brief analysis of these factors. Firstly, much of the research has been carried out in countries other than the UK, which makes it hard to know whether the issues would be the same here. But even more important is the fact that, in some cases, there is nothing that we can really do with the information before the baby is born, other than perhaps stress women unnecessarily.

For example, research by Baker and Barrett (1973), Dillon et al. (1987), Schuchat et al. (1999) and Yagupsky et al. (1991) identified that GBS disease was more likely in babies who weighed less than 2500g at birth. However, while this might be helpful knowledge once a baby is born, we have no really accurate way of predicting birthweight before birth and so there is little we can do with this information. Many babies who are under this birthweight will also be preterm, which is already covered by the RCOG (2012) guidelines.

Dillon et al. (1987) identified prolonged labour as a risk factor, but this study is rather old and based in the US, both of which mean its findings may not be applicable for women giving birth today. In addition, prolonged labour can only be defined as such after the point where antibiotic coverage would have been offered, so it is not particularly helpful. A study by Schuchat et al. (1999) in the USA identified black women, teenage mothers and women who have previously had a miscarriage to be at higher risk. I have been unable to find comparable data relating to UK women, and for this reason I understand the RCOG's hesitancy in recommending antibiotics for more women on the basis of one US study, when the same results weren't found in the UK research. Christensen, et al., (1983) suggested that gestational age more than 42 weeks was a risk factor, which might be of more concern to the RCOG if they didn't already recommend induction of labour before this point (a situation that is discussed in AIMS' book *Inducing Labour: making informed decisions* (Wickham 2014). Finally, Håkansson and Källén (2006) found that women with gestational diabetes were at higher risk but, again, this was not the finding of similar studies which involved UK women and the different definitions of and treatments for gestational diabetes between countries may account for this.

We do not know exactly what percentage of UK women would be offered antibiotics within the current guidelines (that is, if they were followed to the letter in practice), with the only estimate I could find being Oddie and Embleton's (2002) at 16%. The number of women who are deemed to be at risk depends substantially on how many women are deemed to need a swab or urine test for other reasons in pregnancy, and also on the proportion of women who directly request GBS testing, so there will likely always be considerable variation between areas and over time.

Testing for GBS

I have already explained that routine testing for GBS is not recommended in the UK. Some women, however, will have a vaginal swab test that may detect GBS while their midwife or doctor is investigating symptoms of vaginal discharge or irritation. Some women want to be tested for GBS proactively and so they either ask for this to be done on the NHS (which may or may not be successful) or they seek private testing, which at the time of writing costs between £35 and £50. (More details on this can be found in the references and resources at the end of this book). It is also worth noting at this point that some hospitals use more than one of the types of test described below, and it is possible to ask for a more effective test to be carried out.

In this section, I am not going to discuss urine testing for GBS. This is because, although GBS will sometimes be found when urine is tested (e.g. because a woman has a suspected urinary infection), urine testing isn't used to specifically screen for GBS. This is principally because the key issue is whether there is GBS bacteria in the vagina and/or rectum, which is why GBS testing is done on swabs that have been wiped in or near those areas of the body.

There are basically three different types of test for GBS. These are known as the direct plating method (not usually abbreviated), enriched culture medium (ECM) and polymerase chain reaction (PCR) testing. The first two of these tests are also known as culture-based tests, because they involve trying to culture or grow bacteria on a plate on which the swab has been wiped, while PCR testing uses biochemical reactions to identify whether the cells on the swab contain DNA regions that are unique to GBS bacteria. Each of these tests has advantages and disadvantages.

Evaluating screening tests

Any screening test needs to be measured against a number of factors. These include:

1. *Sensitivity,* or how good the test is at picking up a disease (or bacteria) when it is present. Poor sensitivity leads to a high false negative rate, which in the case of GBS would mean that more women who have the bacteria are told they are not carriers and not offered treatment.

2. *Specificity,* which is how good the test is at only identifying people who have the bacteria. Poor specificity leads to a higher false positive rate which leads to more women who do not have the bacteria being told they are carrying it and being offered unnecessary treatment.

3. *Practical considerations;* whether the test can be carried out with the facilities and staff available (for instance, tests requiring

electrical equipment are not feasible in some countries or locations).

4. *Staffing considerations;* who can carry out the test, and whether they need to be specially trained.

5. *Speed of testing;* how long it takes to get a result.

6. *Cost;* some laboratory tests are expensive, and this can make a difference to whether it is feasible to offer the test given the available budget and priorities.

7. *Acceptability of screening method;* whether women are OK with how the sample is collected, tested and the result reported to them.

Each of these has to be balanced up against the others, and in reality most tests in any area of midwifery or medicine have advantages and disadvantages. One last thing to mention before I discuss the specific types of test that are used in an attempt to detect GBS is that, although the term 'gold standard' is sometimes used to describe the test that is considered the best, it is very rare to be certain that a test is 100% effective at determining whether or not a bacteria is present. Because how do we know, and what do we measure it against? We can do research and find that test X picks up more cases than test Y, but although that might be because test X is more sensitive and better at detecting the bacteria than test Y, it might instead be that test X has a high false positive rate. I mention this because all of these tests can only be measured against each other and it is important to remember that, while science, medicine and technology are great tools in our quest for knowledge, they are by no means infallible.

Types of test for GBS

The *direct plating method* was the first form of testing used for GBS bacteria, and is used throughout the UK and many other countries. This kind of test is commonly carried out when a swab is taken and a midwife or doctor sends it to a pathology laboratory to see what bacteria are present in the area that was swabbed. This kind of testing wasn't created specifically to test for GBS, which is one reason that it's not the most accurate test.

When the swab arrives in the laboratory, the laboratory scientist will wipe the swab over a special plate (which you might also know as a petri dish) that contains substances that will encourage the bacteria to grow and/or behave in certain ways. Most culture-based tests use plates which are covered in animal (usually sheep) blood in order to see where certain kinds of bacteria are forming colonies (because they will haemolyse or break down blood – which is why GBS is sometimes called beta haemolytic strep) and then these colonies are tested with chemicals to see if they contain *Streptococcus agalactiae*. Most culture-based tests need to be cultured for 48 hours before a result is available, so the results may not be ready until two or three days after the swab was taken.

The advantages of traditional direct plating testing are that it is relatively cheap and very specific, which means that most of the women identified as having GBS via this test do actually have GBS. However, research studies comparing it with the use of a test involving an enriched culture medium (which I will discuss next) showed that it had low sensitivity. This means that it failed to pick up quite a few women who were shown as having GBS (Nguyen, et al., 1998). The reason for this, and the main problem with the direct plating method, is that other kinds of bacteria can overgrow on the plate and thus mask the existence of GBS (Larsen and Sever, 2008).

In many hospitals in the UK, direct plating is used to test for GBS. However, the accuracy of this test can be enhanced by use of an **enriched culture medium** (ECM). This involves adding a special broth to the plate, which will specifically encourage the growth of GBS (but not other kinds of bacteria) and thus increase the sensitivity of the test and ensure that more of the women who carry GBS are identified through testing.

Again, though, the results take two to three days to be available. Some people have tried to make this faster. For example, Faro et al. (2013) found a way to accelerate culture-based testing, reducing the swab-to-result time to 6.5 hours with comparable accuracy to the existing test, but concluded that this was not without disadvantages and was still unlikely to be fast enough for use when women are in labour.

The cost of ECM testing is also higher than the direct plating method, and another disadvantage is that this test can only look for GBS. This might sound like a rather obvious thing to say, but it is important to remember that the type of test carried out is determined by what the midwife or doctor is looking for. If a swab is being tested to see what bacteria are growing in general, for instance because a woman has symptoms of possible vaginal infection, then a GBS-specific medium isn't useful because it is only going to pick up GBS, and GBS is only one possible cause of the problem. Also, GBS rarely causes infections in adults. But laboratories can't set out lots of different plates for each woman, each looking for a different kind of bacteria, so this is why traditional direct plating tends to be used in this situation. If, however, the test is being carried out specifically to look for GBS, then the use of a GBS-specific ECM is preferable and this is currently considered to be the best test by many people. Because the RCOG (2012) and NICE (2012) do not recommend routine GBS testing however, not all hospitals make this available.

The third kind of testing is completely different and known as **polymerase chain reaction** or PCR testing. Rather than being cultured on a plate over a couple of days, the swabs are placed in a machine which uses biochemical reactions and heat to identify whether or not the cells on the swab contain GBS-related DNA.

PCR testing is not in use in the UK at the time of writing but it has been shown to be more accurate, rapid and practical as an alternative to culture-based testing (Money, et al., 2008, Daniels , et al., 2009, Abdelazim, 2013, Chan, et al., 2014, Håkansson and Källén, 2006, Mueller, et al., 2014). The main barrier is the cost of the equipment needed to undertake PCR testing. In an analysis carried out in Saint-Étienne, France, the PCR test was found to be 'prohibitively expensive' compared to culture-based testing (Poncelet-Jasserand, et al., 2013), although a team led by El Helali et al. (2012) in Paris had calculated this to be cost-neutral in their system. This is not entirely surprising; the cost difference is likely to vary between areas, depending on issues such as the GBS carriage rate, current facilities, staffing levels and the kind of care and interventions that are offered in different circumstances. Economic evaluations of this kind of testing within the context of the UK have found that *"based on their current sensitivity, specificity and cost, screening using rapid tests was dominated by other more cost-effective strategies"* (Kaambwa, et al., 2010).

Rapid PCR testing is increasingly being used on labour wards in areas (outside the UK) which offer all women screening for GBS carriage.

Studies of this have shown that sensitivity and specificity rates are similar between swabs analysed in a laboratory with ECM and on a labour ward via PCR, but more of the samples analysed on the labour ward are likely to be classed as invalid (Håkansson, et al., 2014, Mueller, et al., 2014), which means that they have to be taken again. This was slightly improved by staff training (Mueller, et al., 2014), but labour ward staff are less experienced at this kind of activity than laboratory staff, are often very busy and this is only one of a number of technical processes that they are expected to undertake under pressure. Given the current approach to GBS in the UK, rapid PCR testing is not likely to happen in the foreseeable future.

Availability and timing of testing

Women need to make decisions about whether they want to be screened and/or treated for GBS carriage within the context of what is normally offered in their country or context. I will return to a discussion of the wider issues relating to this decision in part four. The following section looks at the factors that need to be weighed up in situations where women are considering being tested for GBS in pregnancy, either because they are in a country that offers this routinely, or because they are in a country that does not offer it routinely but they are considering whether they might want to pursue this themselves. In this situation, a number of factors need to be weighed up.

1. **What tests are available locally?**

In the UK, some hospitals only offer GBS testing by the direct plating method and, as above, this method is likely to be used if a swab is being tested because a woman is thought to have an infection rather than because the intention is to specifically test for GBS. But in some areas it is the only method offered even when the test is specifically intended to look for GBS. Some hospitals offer ECM testing. In some areas ECM testing is available to all women, but some units will offer ECM testing only under certain circumstances, for instance where particular risk factors exist. Some women have found that their local hospital will carry out an ECM test if specifically asked, but this may not be done routinely or unless specifically requested. As mentioned above, at the time of writing, PCR testing for GBS is not used in the UK, though it is in some other countries. The best way of finding out what is available locally is to ask your midwife or doctor. If they don't know, ask them to put you in touch with somebody who can find out for you. This may be the hospital laboratory itself, or a doctor who works with the laboratory.

2. **Who does the test?**

The RCOG (2012) and NICE (2008) guidance concludes that, as long as they are given appropriate instruction, women are just as good at collecting their own swab as midwives or doctors. Some of the individual studies in this area show that women prefer to collect the swab themselves; while others found that women preferred that a midwife or doctor did the test. I am not going to detail these studies because there is really no question that either of these options are equally good and any woman who decides to have testing should be able to decide which approach is best for her.

3. **Are other tests available privately, at a cost?**

A number of laboratories in the UK offer private ECM testing, either by appointment or by post. When the test is done by post, the laboratory sends out the test kit and the woman does the swab test herself and returns the swabs to the laboratory in special packaging which it provides. The cost of this testing service at the time of writing was around £35-50. The cost of by appointment testing was more variable according to the location and context, but is somewhat higher than this, as it involves having staff members carrying out the swab test. The organisation Group B Strep Support keeps an up-to-date list of laboratories which offer private testing in the UK on its web site at http://gbss.org.uk/what-is-gbs/testing-for-gbs/ecm-test-where-how/ Please also see the resources section for more information on the various groups and facilities relating to GBS information and testing.

4. **What is the best timing for testing?**

It is important not to underestimate the various trade-offs that have to be taken into account if a woman is deciding whether to be tested for GBS using either the direct plating or ECM test. Although the results are sometimes available faster, both of these tests can take 2-3 days to complete, so if a woman wants to know her GBS status before she goes into labour, then she needs to plan to have the test done at least 2-3 days before she is likely to go into labour. This timing is obviously not very easy to predict.

This is one reason why PCR testing is seen as a great advance by some people, although the main downside of this – at least from the point of view of those who make decisions about funding health care – is that it is expensive. One woman who wrote to me from a country which uses PCR testing in labour also mentioned that the speed at which she was tested and told that she was carrying GBS bacteria was quite disconcerting, because she hadn't previously known about this and was suddenly told that she needed antibiotics in labour without having time to properly research this or consider her options.

Making a decision about when to test may be just as crucial as making the decision about whether to test. Very few women will know when they are going to give birth with any real certainty, and even those who know that they will have an induction of labour or a caesarean section on a particular date cannot be sure that they will not go into labour before that date. So if a woman wants to be tested for GBS, then we might imagine that it makes sense to do it sooner rather than later in order to ensure that the result is back before she goes into labour. It is also worth noting that, occasionally, a woman has to be re-tested because a swab didn't contain sufficient material to get a good result, or was lost or contaminated during the testing process. It doesn't happen often but when it does, it means re-swabbing and re-testing, which can take another two or three days.

All of this suggests it makes sense to test as early as possible. But this isn't the easy answer that it might seem, because GBS bacteria are transient – they can come and go – so a woman's GBS status can change. This means that performing the test too long before labour starts increases the chances that the test result will not reflect a woman's actual GBS carrier status when she goes into labour. This can happen in both directions; some of the women who test negative for GBS will be carrying GBS when they are in labour, and they won't be offered antibiotics (unless they are in a country that uses risk-based screening and they have a risk factor), while some of the women who tested positive for GBS will not have this by the time they go into labour, and they will be offered antibiotics.

It is generally accepted that there is no value in doing testing before 35 weeks of pregnancy, as the problem of the rate of change in GBS status between that point and the onset of labour outweighs the likelihood of too many women going into labour before they can have the test.

Also, very few women go into labour before this time . NICE (2008a) recommend that the collection of cultures between 35 and 37 weeks of gestation appears to achieve the best sensitivity and specificity for identifying women who carry GBS at the time of delivery, although this is based on the results of just one study, carried out in the US (Yancey, et al., 1996). Yancey et al. (1996) estimated that the sensitivity of the 35-37 week test for picking up GBS carriage status at birth was 96%, which means that 4% of women who tested negative between 35 and 37 weeks picked up GBS bacteria before they went into labour. However, 13% (about 1 in 8) of the women who tested positive for GBS at 35-37 weeks were not found to have this when tested in labour, although these women would all still have been unnecessarily offered antibiotics.

Studies similar to Yancey et al. (1996) have since been carried out in the Netherlands (Valkenburg-van den Berg, et al., 2006), Thailand (Kovavisarach, et al., 2008) and Portugal (Florindo, et al., 2014), although the tests women may be offered may differ in some way to the testing methods used in all four of these studies. We also don't know whether changes occur in a woman's vagina when she goes into labour that could affect the test results, but I will return to that question below.

Kovavisarach et al.'s (2008) findings agreed with those of Yancey et al. (1996) in that the 35-37 week test results identified 95.4% of women who tested positive for GBS in labour, but the positive predictive value in this study was even poorer. The testing at 35-37 weeks falsely identified an even greater number of women as GBS carriers in labour with only 70.73% of those identified as carrying GBS at 35-37 weeks having a positive test in labour. This means that just under 30% of the women who were identified as carrying GBS at 35-37 weeks were not considered to be carrying it in labour and would have been offered unnecessary antibiotics and/or found that their birth plans might be affected by this. In Valkenburg-van den Berg et al.'s (2006) study, the 35-37 week test wasn't quite as good at identifying women who would have GBS in labour; it correctly identified 93% of the women who had GBS in labour, so 7% of women who had a positive GBS test in labour wouldn't have been offered antibiotics. The positive predictive value was 79%, so in this study 21% of women were deemed to be at risk when they had the test but were not identified as GBS carriers by the time they went into labour.

A more recent study in Portugal by Florindo et al. (2014) compared the results of GBS cultures taken at 35-37 weeks of gestation to the results of GBS cultures in labour and found that 'of 221 prenatally GBS-positive women, only 54 remained positive at delivery, corresponding to a PPV [or positive predictive value] of 24.4%' (Florindo , et al., 2014: 641). In other words, 75.6% of women who were found to be GBS positive at 35-37 weeks of pregnancy were not found to be carrying GBS by the time they gave birth.

This last figure is astonishingly high compared to the results of the other studies just mentioned. The discrepancy may be partially explained by the fact that women in Portugal choose their own laboratory for screening, which meant that the researchers could not confirm the quality of the sampling, swab storage and testing methods that were used in the 35-37 week screening test. Women who are considering private GBS testing may wish to consider this issue and look into what quality control measures are in place in the laboratories that they are considering and whether and how they are regulated.

Florindo et al. (2014) discuss implications for standardisation of GBS detection protocols and screening guidelines, and this may well explain the unusually high results. Even if the magnitude of the difference in Florindo et al.'s (2014) study is unique to their setting, the general trend is not. *'Both negative (NPV) and positive (PPV) predictive values of prenatal GBS cultures relative to the GBS status at delivery are suboptimal, especially the PPV'* (Florindo, et al., 2014: 640). The difference between the antenatal and in-labour rates of GBS carriage in this research also raises an important point for women who are considering getting their own GBS test done about researching the quality of the testing method. The net result of this in all of the studies mentioned here is that, where GBS testing at 35-37 weeks is used as the basis for giving antibiotics in labour, significantly more women will be recommended to have antibiotic treatment than need it.

These findings need to be considered in relation to a number of other factors discussed elsewhere in this book and it is probably inevitable that they are interpreted differently depending on a person's viewpoint. Those who are keen to ensure that they do everything possible to prevent GBS disease and are happy to accept the costs for both mother and baby (which may be physical, emotional and social as well as financial) of administering more antibiotics than necessary tend to be reassured by the relatively high negative predictive value of testing at 35-37 weeks and see this as the best course of action. Those women who want to be tested and perhaps treated but would rather avoid antibiotics and/or potential restrictions to their birth plans unless they can be more certain that their GBS status is accurate may wish to delay testing. Although we know from these studies that somewhere between 13% and 29.27% (or up to 75.6% if we take Florindo et al.'s (2014) figures) of the women identified as being GBS positive at 35-

37 weeks did not test positive for GBS in labour, we don't have any evidence about whether testing at, say, 38 or 39 weeks would be more accurate. This point was also raised by NICE (2008a). We do know, of course, that more women will have gone into labour before that time, so for them the opportunity for testing will have been missed.

As a slight aside, this is where the kind of accelerated testing that Faro et al. (2013) researched could be useful, but this research was not seen as fruitful. It is possible that advances may be made in this area in the future. In addition, and to my knowledge, no-one has researched whether there is a physiological change in GBS status before and/ or during labour. It is possible that there may be a mechanism that prepares a woman's body for labour by 'clearing the way' of bacteria that may be harmful to her baby. Or there may not: my point is that we don't know. We are really only beginning to understand the human microbiome and the importance of bacteria in our lives. If the woman's vagina undergoes changes in order to become more hospitable for the baby to be born, then there is no reason to think that this might not involve changes in the vaginal flora. The existence of a mechanism to reduce GBS bacteria wouldn't necessarily be in conflict with the fact that some babies contract GBS disease. A mechanism to provide protection against potentially harmful bacteria may not work as well in some women, for reasons that may be related to genetics, the stage of pregnancy, the environment, their nutritional and/or immunological status or a combination of these or other factors. This is all, however, completely speculative as no research has been carried out on this question. I mention it because I want to keep pointing out that there are many facets of this topic which have thus far been ignored and which may deserve greater attention.

Screening or no screening?

As you may have gathered from the discussion of the RCOG (2012) guidelines, although the UK doesn't recommend routine screening, many midwives and doctors are fast to recommend, or encourage antibiotics when a woman has been found to carry GBS. This is worth bearing in mind if you are considering whether or not to have screening, especially in view of the previously stated fact that a proportion of women who test positive at 35-37 weeks won't be carrying GBS when they go into labour. I know of at least one case where a woman had a negative GBS test at 39 weeks of pregnancy following a positive test at 37 weeks but was still put under pressure to have antibiotics in labour.

This leads into the second point: once you have a GBS screening test, you can't 'unknow' the results of this, and neither can you remove it from your medical records (Wickham, 2009). Women can find that they are under a lot of pressure to have screening and treatment for GBS – not just from professionals, but sometimes from their family, other women and/or consumer groups – and women may want to think through whether or not they would want treatment before deciding whether or not to have testing.

Many women do not realise that this situation is different from some of the other tests that are offered in pregnancy. With most antenatal screening tests, for instance, you will be offered the option of having a test or not and it will be up to you to make the decision. Your decision will usually be respected either way. In the case of GBS screening, the decision is still up to you, but women in countries which offer universal screening are often put under pressure to accept this, and some women in countries like the UK that use risk-based screening have found that some of the information out there is geared towards persuading them to have a GBS test done privately.

Then, women who have risk factors or who decide to be screened and are found to be GBS positive are often put under significant pressure to have antibiotics in labour. Much of the literature given out on this topic in clinics and hospitals is biased towards having antibiotics and many women have found it to be fear-based rather than informative. As mentioned previously, the decision also has implications in relation to where women are able to give birth, in that they might be refused admission to a birth centre or midwifery-led unit if it does not have facilities for giving intravenous antibiotics, or dealing with the occasional emergency that arises from this. So these are all things to bear in mind as you weigh up the decision that is right for you.

Finally, as the NICE (2008) guideline points out, no research has been carried out to compare antenatal screening with no screening – that is, to see if more babies are saved when women are screened. Nor have any trials been undertaken to compare different screening strategies. As we will discuss in the next section, there are quite a few studies showing correlations (or relationships) between the introduction of GBS-related screening and treatment strategies and a reduction in the number of babies who develop early-onset GBS disease. However, there are a number of things we need to take into consideration when looking at this kind of research and their results may not be as reliable as some people may think.

There are no rights and wrongs here. The important thing is to weigh up the information, consider your own circumstances, beliefs and feelings and to make the best decision that you can for your own personal situation.

Part 3: Explaining the treatment options

While approaches to determining who is at risk differ widely between countries, most maternity care systems have policies clearly stating that, where a baby has been determined to be at risk, the most appropriate response is to offer intravenous antibiotics to the woman during labour. Intravenous antibiotics are thought to help in this situation in two ways. Firstly, it is hoped that they will eliminate the GBS bacteria from the woman's vagina, so that it cannot be transferred to her baby. Secondly, as intravenous antibiotics cross the placenta, they will be in the baby's system when it is born and it is hoped that they may help treat any infection that the baby encounters. But antibiotics come with risks and side effects, and are not for everyone.

Some women who have a risk factor or who have found they carry GBS decide to do nothing except keep a close eye on their baby once she or he is born. Other women decide to have the intravenous antibiotic treatment offered within systems of maternity care, while others use alternative approaches in an attempt to treat this. The current recommendation from the RCOG, (2012) is that:

> "For women who have accepted IAP, benzylpenicillin should
> be administered as soon as possible after the onset of labour
> and given regularly until delivery. Clindamycin should be
> administered to those women allergic to benzylpenicillin.

> It is recommended that 3 g intravenous benzylpenicillin be
> given as soon as possible after the onset of labour and 1.5 g
> 4-hourly until delivery. Clindamycin 900 mg should be given
> intravenously 8-hourly to those allergic to benzylpenicillin."
> (RCOG, 2012: 5)

Before I look at the evidence and other issues relating to antibiotics, I want to explain what having antibiotics in labour entails for a woman who decides to take this path. Apart from anything else, this enables me to define and explain some of the terminology at the outset.

When women decide to have antibiotics in labour

If a woman decides to have antibiotics in labour, these will be given directly into her bloodstream (intravenously) through a plastic tube (cannula) which is inserted into a vein in her hand. Although it is possible to get oral antibiotics (which are taken into the mouth as tablets), these are not considered to be effective enough in the case of GBS. We will consider whether intravenous antibiotics are effective below. The cannula (also called a venflon) will be inserted by a midwife or doctor by means of a special needle which is removed as soon as the tube has been inserted.

The cannula is usually inserted once the woman is considered to be in established labour. ('Established labour' is the frustrating term used by midwives and doctors to describe when they think that the woman's labour has reached the point where they feel it is going to carry on until the baby is born. This can feel confusing and frustrating for women because it doesn't account for the hours of labour that she may have experienced before this point, and it is one of those definitions which have little meaning within the more important context of the woman's experience.) One exception to this is where a woman is having her labour induced. In this situation, the first dose of antibiotics will usually be given at the onset of the Syntocinon drip which is used to stimulate contractions (see Wickham, 2014). This is especially the case where women have already had one or more babies, and this is done to increase the chance that the antibiotics will be given at least four hours before the baby is born.

A skilled midwife or doctor can usually insert a cannula quickly, although it can be painful, especially as it may be difficult for the woman to stay still if she is experiencing pain. Also, some practitioners prefer to use a fairly large cannula in case it is needed in an emergency situation later. If a woman decides to have antibiotics but does not like needles, she may wish to let her midwife know this. The woman might want to request that a smaller cannula is used and that this procedure is performed by someone who is skilled and experienced.

In some areas, a blood sample is taken when the cannula is inserted, most often as a precautionary measure in case the woman needs a blood transfusion later. Women can ask what this blood will be tested for and let the midwife or doctor know if they do not wish for this to happen. As with any intravenous procedure, there is a risk of infection from the cannula site, although this is rare. Other risks of having intravenous antibiotics are discussed on page 95-98.

The antibiotics are usually prescribed by a doctor and usually given by a midwife, but this may differ in some areas. There are two main ways of giving the antibiotics; the first dose is usually put in a small bag of saline fluid which is hung up on something like a drip pole or machine while it drips down into the woman's arm through the cannula. The second and subsequent doses can be put in a syringe and given by slow injection directly into the cannula in the woman's arm. This is sometimes referred to as a bolus.

When giving the first dose of antibiotics, the midwife or doctor will usually inject the antibiotic solution into a small bag of saline fluid. They will then push one end of a long plastic tube into the bag of antibiotic solution and attach the other end to the cannula, using a special clip or machine to control the rate at which the antibiotic drips into the woman's hand through the cannula. The first recommended dose of antibiotics for GBS treatment usually takes about 15 to 20 minutes to drip through. With this method, it usually takes about five minutes for the drugs to be slowly injected into the cannula, and then the syringe can be removed and the cannula bandaged as before.

Because the RCOG (2012) recommendation is that antibiotics continue to be given throughout labour, at four or six-hourly intervals until the baby is born, the cannula will usually be left in for the whole of the woman's labour. It should not be continually attached to a drip, though, unless intravenous fluids are being given for other reasons (for instance because the woman has an epidural, or her labour has been induced or augmented (artificially speeded up) with a drug such as Syntocinon). If the woman does not have a drip, the cannula should be carefully taped or bandaged in place once the first dose of antibiotic has been given so that the woman can move freely without fearing that she will bang or catch the cannula on something and hurt her hand or dislodge the cannula. If the woman wants to have a shower, bath or use a birth pool, a glove and bandage can be used to keep her hand and the IV site dry.

If it has only been used for antibiotics (and not other fluids or drugs) and the woman has not had any problems (such as excessive bleeding) the cannula will usually be removed as soon as the woman has given birth. Some women are asked to wait until they have been to the toilet and/or are ready to shower, but a woman can ask for it to be removed at any time. The cannula needs to be removed carefully, as it is in vein which may bleed, and it will need to have pressure put on it for a short while after it is removed. It is not uncommon to have a bruise on an IV site for a few days afterwards, and it may be tender.

Having a cannula in place does not mean that a woman should be denied access to a pool for labour and/or birth.

Local variation in antibiotic treatment

While the RCOG (2012) recommend that benzylpenicillin is the antibiotic of choice, with clindamycin as the alternative where women who decide to have antibiotics are allergic to penicillin, these are not always the antibiotics that are offered in practice. In fact, there are a number of areas in which local protocols frequently differ from the RCOG (2012) guidance, and this is one of them. While I have been writing this book I have been asking UK midwives and doctors what the policy is in their area, and a surprising number have told me that their unit policy differs from the RCOG (2012) and NICE (2012) guidance. The most common examples of variation that I encountered include that:

- The primary antibiotic used to treat women who are GBS positive and who decide to have antibiotics is not penicillin but gentamicin. Most frequently, 3g of this is initially given as an infusion, with subsequent doses of 1.5g via bolus.

- The antibiotic given to women who decide to have antibiotics but have a penicillin allergy is not clindamycin but erythromycin. Erythromycin is usually given 8 hourly, which has implications if there is a local assumption that a woman is only covered if she has had two doses of antibiotics in labour. This is because some paediatricians strongly recommend that, if women have not received two doses of antibiotic in labour, their baby should be admitted to the special care unit and receive intravenous antibiotics. But some women – especially those having second or subsequent babies – may not be in labour long enough to be given a second dose.

- There is also occasional variation in the local dosage and frequency of administration of the recommended antibiotics benzylpenicillin and clindamycin. For example, in some areas 800mg of clindamycin is given 6 hourly rather than 900mg 8 hourly. In reality, these are not that different when you compare dosage over time, and the thinking may be that a woman is more likely to get a second dose before she gives birth, but the deviation from the guideline is still worth noting because women who decide they want to have antibiotics may wish to ask about what antibiotics would be recommended ahead of time.

The RCOG (2012) itself notes that *'dosage regimens are based on tradition rather than evidence'*, which may also explain some of these differences. Despite these deviations, most local guidelines are clear that broad spectrum antibiotics such as ampicillin should be avoided where possible. This is because the overuse of antibiotics, and especially broad spectrum antibiotics, is causing certain kinds of bacteria to become resistant to the antibiotics, and there is a need to save these for situations when they are needed to treat babies who have an actual infection rather than overusing them as a preventative measure.

Antibiotics: the dimensions of effectiveness

Probably the most important question that we need to consider in this section of the book is: do antibiotics work? That is, are they effective at preventing GBS disease in babies?

Unfortunately, the answer to that isn't as straightforward as we might like, as I will explain over the next few pages, but if I had to summarise what we currently know at this point in time in three words, they would be: *we don't know.*

The reason we don't know is that we don't have good enough research data. The reason we don't have good enough research data is that we haven't run large enough trials of appropriate quality to be able to effectively measure the effectiveness of antibiotics against GBS disease. This situation is summarised by the authors of the largest and best-respected medical review in this area:

> *"Ideally the effectiveness of IAP to reduce neonatal GBS infections should be studied in adequately sized double-blind controlled trials. The opportunity to conduct such trials has likely been lost, as practice guidelines (albeit without good evidence) have been introduced in many jurisdictions."* (Ohlsson and Shah, 2014: 1)

In other words, we don't have good evidence from clinical trials that antibiotics work but these are still offered to women whose babies are perceived to be at risk of GBS disease because this has become the standard of care despite the lack of evidence. A full explanation of why this is the case is beyond the scope of this book, but much of the reason for this relates to the way our culture views health, responsibility and what people can expect from midwives, doctors and systems of health care. Some practitioners feel that they would rather do something (even if it's not necessarily effective and even if it has side effects) than nothing, and some parents feel the same way. Some practitioners are scared that they might be sued if they don't do everything possible, even if there isn't good evidence to support it. Once you have a few people doing something (like recommending antibiotics because a baby is deemed to be at risk from GBS) it soon becomes a norm and an expectation. It is then difficult for professionals not to recommend it, as they tend to be judged against what most other professionals do as well as what the evidence says.

That said, there are a few studies of lesser quality that indicate that antibiotics are effective at reducing GBS carriage, but I will return to a discussion of those in a moment. First, I want to explain more about the review above, which entails a brief discussion about how we measure the effectiveness of medical treatments.

Measuring effectiveness in research_

There are lots of different ways in which research can be undertaken, and all have their place, but if you want to measure the effectiveness of a drug at treating a particular disease, then it is very well accepted within science and medicine that the best way to do this is by carrying out a randomised controlled trial. In this kind of study, you take a group of people, randomly divide them into two (or sometimes more) groups, and give one group the treatment and the other group a placebo that looks, smells, tastes and feels like the treatment. Then you see what happens in each group. The reason for having a placebo is because, when someone gives us a pill, sometimes we get better because we think we will get better – this is called the placebo effect – and in the ideal trial neither the woman or her caregiver knows who has the real drug and who has the placebo. When a placebo is used in this way, it is called a double blind trial (because neither the woman nor her midwife or doctor knows who is having the real drug).

In this kind of trial, we need to be very clear and specific about what we think the drug will do and have a very measureable outcome. For instance - and I apologise for the starkness of this, but it is the reality of medical research – we might decide we are going to count the number of babies who die or who suffer from a particular problem after getting a disease. The researchers also need to be very clear about how a disease is defined and diagnosed. We have already seen that testing isn't 100% accurate, and the symptom pictures of different diseases can often look similar, so all of these things need to be considered very carefully. Also, because diseases such as GBS disease are thankfully rare, a research study that was going to include mortality (death) as an outcome would need to randomise an awful lot of women and babies in order to see whether there was a difference between the treatment and the placebo.

Hopefully, that brief explanation of the complexities of a research trial will go part of the way to explain why it is not always straightforward to find the answer to questions such as whether antibiotics are effective at reducing the mortality rate from GBS disease. But let's look at the review of the trials that have been carried out in this area and apply this, as that will explain more.

The Cochrane review

The Cochrane Collaboration has published several versions of a review of the trials which have been carried out *'to assess the effect of intrapartum antibiotics for maternal Group B haemolytic streptococci (GBS) colonization on mortality from any cause, from GBS infection and from organisms other than GBS'* (Ohlsson and Shah 2014: 1). The authors describe the importance of reviewing the trials in this area thus:

> *"It is important to know if intrapartum antibiotics do more*
> *good than harm in trying to reduce mortality and morbidity*

from neonatal GBS infections. Most women colonized with GBS are asymptomatic [without symptoms of infection], so screening is necessary if these women are to be identified. However, of the women in labor who are GBS positive, very few will give birth to babies who are infected with GBS. Hence, giving IV antibiotics to all women in labor who are GBS positive will put a large number of women and babies at risk of adverse effects unnecessarily. These adverse effects include potentially fatal anaphylaxis, increase in drug-resistant organisms and the medicalization of labor and the neonatal period (RCOG 2003)." (Ohlsson and Shah, 2014: 4).

Ohlsson and Shah (2014) set out to see if antibiotics worked for _known_ group B strep colonisation. I am emphasising this because I want to highlight the slipperiness of the word 'know' in this situation. We might say that only women who live in countries like the US or Australia which offer routine screening and women who actively choose to have GBS screening will _know_ if they carry GBS or not. But we have to bear in mind that the tests aren't totally accurate, and that GBS carriage status may change. Aside from these concerns, however, the review didn't set out to look at the effectiveness of antibiotics in countries like the UK and New Zealand which offer antibiotics when women have risk factors. Women in countries using risk-based screening aren't really at a disadvantage here, though. Despite searching on a global scale, Ohlsson and Shah (2014) identified only four relevant randomised controlled trials which met their criteria for the review. Many more trials have been carried out, but these were rejected for one or more reasons.

The trials that were included in the review were published between 1986 and 2002. Three of the included trials, involving a total of 500 women, evaluated the effect of antibiotics versus no antibiotics. However, none of these used blinding, and for this and several other reasons they were considered to be at high risk for potential bias: that is, their findings were not necessarily reliable. The fourth trial, involving a total of 352 women, compared two different antibiotics: penicillin and ampicillin. It is not clear whether women and their caregivers were blinded to which antibiotic they had and this trial was considered to be of better quality than the other three, but as it did not include a control group of women who did not have an antibiotic, its results aren't that useful in relation to the question of whether antibiotics are more effective than not having antibiotics.

Ohlsson and Shah (2014) went on to analyse and present the results of the trials, although they repeatedly point out that they do not consider the data to be trustworthy because the trials were flawed:

> *"The use of IAP did not significantly reduce the incidence of all cause mortality, mortality from GBS infection or from infections caused by bacteria other than GBS. The incidence of early GBS infection was reduced with IAP compared to no treatment (risk ratio (RR) 0.17, 95% confidence interval (CI) 0.04 to 0.74, three trials, 488 infants; risk difference -0.04, 95% CI -0.07 to -0.01; number needed to treat to benefit 25, 95% CI 14 to 100, I^2 0%)." (Ohlsson and Shah , 2014: 1-2).*

In lay terms this means that the antibiotics seemed to decrease the number of babies who developed GBS infection (although we mustn't forget that the doctors diagnosing GBS infection would have known whether women had the antibiotics or not, which could have subconsciously affected their assessment) but the antibiotics made no difference to the numbers of babies who died, whether from GBS or another infection.

The small numbers of women included in the trials makes it rather unlikely that this data would show a difference in mortality anyway, and this is one of the things that Ohlsson and Shah (2014) have to say about the untrustworthiness of these findings:

"It is remarkable that in North America the commonly implemented practice of IAP to GBS colonized women has been so poorly studied. Only three randomized controlled trials conducted more than 20 years ago in three different countries and enrolling a total of 500 women have been published. We identified serious concerns of bias in these trials affecting our ability to draw conclusions from this systematic review. Concerns include no preset sample sizes, the lack of a placebo in the control groups, women and care-providers not blinded to group assignment, reporting on outcomes while the trials were ongoing, and exclusion of women who developed signs of infections in labor." (Ohlsson and Shah, 2014: 14)

Understandably, this situation leaves many parents and practitioners feeling confused and frustrated. There is no good randomised trial data to show us whether antibiotics have any effect on reducing the number of babies who die or become sick from early-onset GBS disease. There is a desperate need for good randomised controlled trials in this area, because we genuinely don't know whether antibiotics work to reduce mortality (death) and/or morbidity (illness) from GBS disease or not. However, the entrenched nature of obstetric practices such as this within a risk-focused culture mean that many people perceive it as next to impossible to run the research trials that would generate this knowledge. But the alternative to running these trials is to continue to recommend a treatment which we hope might work but whose effectiveness is actually unknown and which we do know can be harmful.

Other research on antibiotics and GBS carriage

A significant number of other studies have been carried out and published in this area, and I will look at some of their results here, but it is important to reiterate that most of these are not randomised controlled trials, and thus are not the best kind of research to use to evaluate the effectiveness of a treatment. (I am not going to look further at the randomised controlled trials that Ohlsson and Shah (2014) rejected from their analysis, because they are of even less use in answering our questions than those already discussed).

The reason that these other kinds of studies are not ideal is because there are so many places where bias can enter the frame, which can mean that the results and any conclusions we draw from the results might be wrong. Any kind of knowledge, including that derived from research findings, needs to be considered in context, and in this section I will offer a bit more contextual information about what we can and cannot learn from different kinds of studies.

Ohlsson and Shah (2014: 4) offer a good overview of the state of the rest of the science:

> "Although these current guidelines are based on studies of poor quality (Ohlsson 1994), there seems to be a temporal association between the introduction of guidelines and a decline in the GBS EOD [early onset disease] rate (CDC 2005; CDC 2007; Schrag 2002). The incidence of invasive early-onset GBS disease decreased from 1.8 cases/1000 live

births in the early 1990s to 0.26 cases/1000 live births in 2010 (Schrag 2013). However, there has been no reduction in LOD [or late onset] GBS disease in infants (CDC 2007; Schrag 2013). Mortality has decreased. The same literature has been interpreted differently by different professional organizations. All cases of EOD cannot be prevented."

The fact that the literature has been interpreted differently in different areas is very telling, as it reflects the way in which the research findings are not clear-cut. The study by Schrag et al. (2002), for instance, is often quoted by groups promoting screening and treatment for GBS carriage. This was a large retrospective cohort study, and these researchers concluded that screening (and, as a consequence, antibiotic treatment) reduced the rate of GBS disease overall, although they measured the effectiveness of this to be in the region of 86-89%, so a proportion of babies still got GBS disease despite their mothers having had the recommended screening and/or antibiotics in labour.

But there is an important distinction between association (or correlation) and causation. Many researchers find, when they analyse their data, that two things appear to increase at the same time. Or maybe one thing appears to increase at the same time as another thing decreases, but they seem to change at the same time, so we say that they may be associated, or correlated (literally co-related). When studies show what appear to be correlations, it is very tempting to conclude that one of them causes the other – which is where we get the term causation. The temptation is even greater if it already seems plausible that these things are related and/or if the research concerns a question which is highly emotive – such as whether something can save the lives of babies.

I want to be very clear here. I am not saying that antibiotics don't help. I am saying that, from a scientific perspective, the research that has been done to date unfortunately isn't good enough to tell us for sure whether they help or not or, if they do help, how much difference they make. It is, again, pretty clear that they are not 100% effective. The only kind of research that can tell us whether two things are genuinely related – and thus whether antibiotics are truly effective – are those randomised controlled trials. In such studies, all the other variables are held constant and the only thing that varies is the one being studied. Just as importantly, nobody should know who is having the antibiotic and who is having the placebo in order that we can ensure that people's preconceptions and other psychological aspects like the placebo effect aren't going to affect the care that women and babies receive and thus potentially bias the results.

As Ohlsson and Shah (2014) noted, the opportunity for good research in this area has all but been lost because the idea that antibiotics work and should be offered to women deemed to be at risk has become so accepted in practice. A recent study by Eastwood et al. (2014) looked at the situation in Ireland by means of a retrospective cohort study. Their findings were interesting in that, while they clearly perceive antibiotics to be the best course of action, they also found (like Schrag, et al., 2002) that giving antibiotics in labour doesn't prevent all cases of GBS disease, which could be taken to mean that we need more and better research in order to better understand what is going on here. But often the best we can do these days is to look at how closely the guidelines are followed because, again, it is deemed unethical by some to have those control groups of women not having antibiotics in order to see if those antibiotics work.

A number of studies have looked at whether giving antibiotics reduces the chance that a woman has GBS in or around her vagina, on the basis that this is considered a surrogate measure of antibiotic effectiveness. The researchers argue from their findings that antibiotics such as penicillin (McNanley, et al., 2007) and clindamycin (Knight, et al., 2012) reduce the rate of vaginal GBS carriage in women who are carrying GBS. Both of these studies involved taking several swabs from the vaginas of relatively small numbers of women (50 and 21 respectively) who were receiving antibiotics during their labour and seeing if the colony count (or the amount of GBS bacteria found on each successive swab) decreased. It did, and it seems plausible to think that antibiotics have this effect, but again the researchers didn't study a control group of women who didn't have antibiotics. This means that we don't know what would have happened to those women by comparison or, if antibiotics do help, how great the effect is. Both of these things would be useful for women to be able to take into account when they make decisions about GBS.

What about measuring what happens to babies in the real world? Research by Turrentine et al. (2013) showed that babies whose mothers had more than 4 hours of antibiotic treatment in labour were less likely to be admitted to a special care unit and/or be diagnosed as having an infection than babies whose mothers had less than 4 hours of antibiotic treatment. This also seems to be suggestive of antibiotics being helpful. But in this case what we don't know is whether some of the decisions to admit these babies or diagnose and treat them for infection were made *because* the women had had fewer than four hours of antibiotic treatment. In this study, the diagnosis of sepsis was made on the basis of clinical signs, which are arguably more subjective than the results of tests – although, as we saw in the previous section, tests are not always accurate either. It might be that doctors were concerned about these babies because they already perceived that it was important to treat women for more than four hours. I certainly know of many paediatricians who will recommend admitting and treating babies who are considered to be at risk for GBS but whose mothers did not receive four hours' worth of antibiotics, for instance because their labour was short.

It is hard to know how to summarise this area in a helpful way. There are a decent number of nationally-recognised studies such as those by the CDC (2005, 2007) and Schrag et al. (2002) that many people are happy to cite as proof that antibiotics work. The data generated within these studies do seem to show that the rate of GBS has come down since we started to screen and treat women, which suggests that antibiotics may work on a population basis. And the trials show that antibiotics reduce the chance of babies becoming colonised with GBS. But it is important to remember that major studies (Schrag, et al., 2002, Eastwood, et al., 2014) show that antibiotics do not help in all cases and that none of these studies are of the quality needed to properly evaluate the effectiveness of antibiotic treatment to prevent GBS disease. There is an awful lot about this area that we do not know or fully understand.

Some people and organisations cite the results of some of the studies that I have discussed here as if they were unequivocal or undoubted fact, while others do not want to take the received view at face value, and this is why I have gone into some depth in this section. The fact that there aren't any decent randomised controlled trials in this area is a huge problem, and not just from the point of view of not wanting to over-intervene or medicalise women's labours, or because of concern about antibiotic resistance. If we think we already have the answer and thus see antibiotics as the only or best solution, we may miss other possible ways of dealing with the problem of GBS disease. These other ways might include knowledge that could help narrow down the numbers of babies who are 'at risk' and/or other treatments which could help to reduce that risk. It is important not to forget that doing nothing is often a very reasonable option as well, especially when our knowledge in and of an area is questionable and the treatment carries unwanted side effects.

If antibiotics, then which one, and for how long?

I have already discussed the antibiotics recommended in the UK, but I want to return to this briefly to note that some antibiotics are more controversial than others. Co-amoxiclav is not recommended because of an association with neonatal necrotising enterocolitis (a disease in which parts of the bowel are damaged, sometimes severely) in the ORACLE trial (Kenyon, et al., 2001). Vancomycin is the subject of ongoing debate in the medical journals. It is considered inappropriate for the treatment of GBS carriage in some areas because there is a perceived need to reserve it for women who really need it, rather than allowing resistance to this to develop with overuse (Pelaez, et al., 2009). It has also been found not to be effective by Onwuchuruba et al. (2014), but the principles on which this assertion was based were then challenged in a letter by Tse and Wong (2014), to which the authors responded, thus continuing a discussion about effectiveness versus resistance (Towers, et al., 2014). The existence of so much disagreement and debate in the medical literature is not very helpful to women, although that is a function of the state of the science and not the fault of those involved in the debate.

At the time of publication of the RCOG (2012) guidelines, current clindamycin resistance rates in England and Wales were 10%. This is the percentage of cases where the antibiotic will not have any effect against the bacteria because the bacteria have developed resistance to the antibiotic. These rates also differ among countries, for instance Shore and Yudin (2012) found the clindamycin resistance rate to be 19% and the erythromycin resistance rate to be 22% in a region of Canada. The problem of antibiotic resistance is why the antibiotics of choice vary between areas, as also discussed in a recent paper by Schrag and Verani (2013). These rates are likely to keep going up the more we use antibiotics but, again, the results need to be treated with caution.

In most areas, four hours' worth of antibiotics in labour is recommended. The origin of this appears to be partly traditional, but it has been widely adopted and is the basis of many of the research studies. The four-hour theory was briefly challenged by Barber et al. (2008), who measured the level of antibiotic (penicillin) in the cord blood of babies born to women who had antibiotic treatment in labour. They found that the levels of antibiotic in babies' blood increased over the first hour (that they were given to the baby's mother) but then decreased. This meant that babies who were born before their mothers had had four hours of antibiotic coverage actually had more antibiotics in their systems than babies who were born after their mother had more than four hours of antibiotics. However, more recent studies (Fairlie, et al., 2013, Turrentine, et al., 2013), have shown that the relationship between the antibiotic concentration in fluids such as blood and the effects of this on bacteria is rather more complex than thought (Turrentine, 2014). Most practitioners continue to recommend four hours' worth, and in many areas if a woman does not receive two doses of intravenous antibiotics then she may be advised to consent to her baby having intravenous antibiotics, which I shall discuss in part four.

The risks of antibiotics

On a global scale, antibiotic resistance is one of the most concerning risks of using antibiotics, especially in large numbers of woman and/ or babies (Ledger, 2006, Barcaite, et al., 2008, Singleton 2007, Joachim, et al., 2009, Lee, et al., 2010, Shore and Yudin, 2012, Schrag and Verani, 2013, Seale and Millar, 2014). Below, I will discuss how this is a problem for individuals. No-one wants to put babies at unnecessary risk, but the irony is that one of the most significant consequences of current screening and treatment programmes which involve giving antibiotics to large numbers of labouring women whose babies are deemed to be at risk of disease (which is different from definitely having disease) may be that future generations will not have effective antibiotics even for babies who are diagnosed with actual disease.

Another potentially enormous but unquantifiable problem relates to an area that we are only just beginning to understand. I began this book by discussing the relationships between humans and bacteria, and scientists have started to use terms such as the human microbiome in order to discuss the range of microorganisms that live on and within our bodies. Recent research is suggesting that not only are bacteria beneficial, but they need to be passed on to the baby during birth via its mother's vagina and have an important part to play in future health, especially relating to the gut and digestion, but in many other areas of wellbeing as well (Turnbaugh, et al., 2007, Collado, et al., 2012). Scientists and researchers are concerned about the potential risks to antibiotic overuse both in general (Blaser, 2011) and to the baby whose mother receives antibiotics in labour (Neu, 2007, Broe, et al., 2014). This latter concern is supported by the research showing that one of the risks of caesarean section is that these bacteria do not get passed on, which can lead to problems in babies (Grönlund, et al., 1999, Blaser, 2011).

The problems arise because antibiotics are not particularly selective, and many beneficial bacteria will be killed by them, which may have considerable but as yet unquantified knock-on effects in both women and babies (Stokholm, et al., 2013). Antibiotics can create changes in women's and babies' gut bacteria and faecal flora which can cause gastro-intestinal problems and these changes might be permanent (Ambrose, et al., 1985) and they have been associated with an increased chance of postnatal yeast infection in women and babies (Dinsmoor, et al., 2005). We need more research into this area. Several women who contacted me while I was writing this book anecdotally reported their concern that their babies had developed gut problems after they had agreed to have antibiotics in labour in an attempt to reduce the risk of GBS disease. Another woman mentioned that her baby's cord had taken far longer to fall off than she expected from previous experience, and she wondered if this was due to a lack of normal bacteria after he had been given antibiotics. Possible associations like these need to be investigated.

Some of the more common but less severe side effects of antibiotics include disturbances to the digestive system including bloating, indigestion, feeling or being sick and/or having diarrhoea. NHS Choices (2014) estimate that around 1 in 10 people who take antibiotics experience this, and they estimate that around 1 in 15 people have a mild allergic reaction.

Intravenous antibiotics can also cause severe allergic reactions in women, which can also pose a threat to the unborn baby (Dunn , et al., 1999, Jao, et al., 2006, Khan, et al., 2008, Berthier, et al., 2007, Chaudhuri, et al., 2008). This is a rare occurrence, and is estimated to occur in between 1 and 10000 and 1 in 2000 cases (NHS Choices, 2014), but the consequences can be very serious, which is one reason why many practitioners are reluctant to give intravenous antibiotics at home or in a community setting. Previous tolerance of any or a particular kind of intravenous antibiotic offers a degree of reassurance but is not a guarantee of safety.

Antibiotics can affect the baby's immune system which in turn can increase the chance of the baby being susceptible to other bacteria, e.g. ampicillin resistant *Enterobacteriaceae* (Edwards, et al., 2002, Bedford Russell and Murch, 2006). Other potential effects on the baby's immune system were identified in studies by Glasgow et al. (2007) and Ashkenazi-Hoffnung et al (2011), who found that antibiotics given in labour increased the incidence of later bacterial infections in infants. Given the enormity of this problem, we have a scarcity of research and a recent review of this topic by Seale and Millar (Seale and Millar, 2014) concluded that more work is needed in this area.

Diseases such as asthma (Kozyrskyj, et al., 2011), allergy (Kozyrskyj, et al., 2011), childhood obesity (Ajslev, et al., 2011) and obsessive compulsive disorder (Rees, 2014) have been associated with early exposure to antibiotics. As with the discussion about the effectiveness of antibiotics above, I want to point out that much of this research shows association rather than causation and far more work is needed to confirm these concerns.

There are other risks of antibiotic use noted in the literature, although as these involve giving antibiotics in pregnancy rather than labour they are not a problem in relation to GBS prevention if the current RCOG (2012) guidance is followed. Andersen et al. (2013) identified a possible link between antibiotic use in early pregnancy and miscarriage.

Finally, although this is not a direct risk of antibiotic usage per se, it would be remiss of me not to mention somewhere that the choice of birth environment may play a significant part in shaping the experience of woman and baby. There are risks to going into hospital to give birth, including a greater likelihood of having interventions and being exposed to bacteria and other infective agents. The risks in the list above need to be considered in the context of the environment in which the woman will give birth and in which the baby will spend his or her first few days, and I will look at this more closely in the next section. In relation to the risks of antibiotics, however, Eastwood et al. (2014: 6) sum up the situation rather succinctly when they write that: *"Ultimately, the long-term effects of antibiotic use in pregnancy on the infant are not known."*

GBS, antibiotics and place of birth

As mentioned on several occasions previously, one of the most significant risks of having GBS screening and/or treatment is the way in which this can lead to limitations being placed on where the woman can give birth and on what care and treatment she can access. This is not just when women decide to decline antibiotic treatment, but also when they decide to have antibiotics but are told that they can only get this treatment in certain places.

Let me say firstly that no-one can deny a woman the right to give birth at home if that is what she chooses. But if a woman who carries

GBS wants to give birth at home and have intravenous antibiotics in labour, she may be told that this is not possible. There are a couple of reasons that Trusts are reluctant to facilitate women having intravenous antibiotics at home. These include that:

- Antibiotics are powerful drugs and allergic reactions are possible, so it is considered better to give them in a setting with fast access to emergency facilities, drugs and equipment.

- Local protocol generally dictates that drugs that will be given intravenously need to be checked by two registered professionals (e.g. midwives) in order to ensure accuracy and safety and reduce the chance of drug errors, yet usually only one midwife is present at a woman's home until she nears the end of her labour. Sending a second midwife in order to check drugs would have implications for the care of other women, especially where there are staff shortages.

AIMS and I do know of situations where a woman has been given intravenous antibiotics at home, after long discussion with a Supervisor of Midwives about the benefits and risks of this and the creation of an individualised plan of care, but these instances are rare. It may be possible to negotiate this, but denying women intravenous antibiotics at home is not analogous to some of the other situations we encounter in which women are told they cannot make certain decisions. Serious concerns about giving intravenous antibiotics at home exist in the district nursing profession and amongst other community-based professionals, and often patients will only be given intravenous antibiotics at home if they have previously and recently had the same dose of the same antibiotic in hospital. This is because it is then known that they haven't had an allergic reaction before, although even this is not a guarantee that they will not have a reaction. District nurses who give intravenous antibiotics at home have to undergo additional training in dealing with anaphylactic (allergic) reactions, and most midwives have not undertaken this training and nor do they carry the drugs needed to reverse a potential emergency.

For all these reasons, while some women have been able to negotiate this, it is not straightforward. I know of instances where a woman wanting a home birth and intravenous antibiotics went to the hospital in early labour, had antibiotics, and then went home. In at least one case, clindamycin was given instead of benzylpenicillin because the woman did not intend to attend hospital to have a second dose and the coverage was thought to last longer for than for benzylpenicillin.

If women who have decided to give birth in a birth centre or midwifery-led unit are found to carry GBS, they may be told that they cannot give birth there. The most common reasons given for this are that the units do not have the facilities to deal with emergencies arising from the administration of antibiotics (as above) or that the units do not have the facilities or staff to care for or observe babies born to women who carry GBS. This presents a stark choice: the woman can either go to the hospital to give birth, or she can stay at home but (as above) she will be unlikely to get antibiotics if that is what she would want. However, this varies considerably in different areas, and it is best to find out what would happen locally, ideally before you decide whether or not to have screening. This is because it is not possible to 'un-know' your GBS carriage status and you may find that this knowledge changes professionals' perceptions of what your options are (Wickham, 2009).

Women who decide that they do not want to have antibiotics may also wish to consider the kind of care they would receive in different settings as a result of this choice. Again, women who have been found to carry GBS and who go to hospital may find that they are put under considerable pressure to accept antibiotics. If they decline antibiotics, as I will discuss in part four, they may find that they are under pressure to allow antibiotics to be given to their baby.

Other possible treatments

A number of alternative remedies and treatments have been used by women in an attempt to either reduce GBS colonization and/ or reduce the risk of GBS disease. I make the distinction between the two because AIMS and I am well aware that a few women turn to alternative treatments not so much because they feel concerned about the risk of GBS disease in their babies, but because they find themselves in a situation where they feel unable to decline GBS testing and want to try and increase the chance that the test is negative. In one example this was because a woman was told that a negative test was essential before she would be able to give birth in a midwifery-led unit). This is a shocking indictment of the maternity services, and AIMS is always there to support women who need support on such matters.

I want to briefly mention that some women and caregivers have used or considered oral or intramuscular antibiotics rather than intravenous antibiotics. This has mainly been in situations where a woman wants to give birth at home or has a severe needle phobia. We have very little knowledge about whether these are useful. A study by Gardner et al. in (1979) showed oral antibiotics to be ineffective against GBS, and they have rarely been considered in relation to GBS since, although the RCOG (2012) also notes that they are variably absorbed in labour. In addition, these are prescription drugs in many countries, so the situations in which women have taken these have usually been rather unusual ones involving the collaboration of a health care professional.

Much of what we can say to summarise the other approaches in this area is similar to what I have said in relation to intraveouous antibiotics. As with antibiotics, we don't have good enough research to know whether most of these alternative treatments work. Some people swear by one or more of these (as with antibiotics) but their knowledge isn't based on good randomised controlled trial evidence. Because the main focus of alternative remedies (like with antibiotics) is to clear the vagina and/or rectum of GBS bacteria, they may also disrupt the normal flora of the vagina. Alternative remedies may carry a risk of local reaction or inflammation, as with antibiotics. Most of these remedies, however, do not carry the same risks of anaphylaxis or potential antibiotic resistance and I have not come across any association between the remedies discussed below and particular diseases, but I will discuss any specific concerns as I go through the various treatments which have been proposed.

Vaginal Douching

Vaginal douching is an often-discussed treatment for reducing vaginal GBS carriage. It has long been known that vaginal douching can cause a transient reduction of vaginal bacteria. Most of this effect is likely to be due to the simple act of washing the surface of the vagina, but the use of certain substances can further increase the reduction in bacterial numbers (Onderdonk, et al., 1992). In a very small study that evaluated the effect of using douche preparations for various periods of time, Onderdonk et al. (1992) found that douche preparations containing acetic acid or povidone-iodine were more effective at reducing bacterial count than when the same women used physiologic saline (salt water). By contrast, a Turkish study by Sakru et al. (2006) found that women who used soap for daily vaginal douching were more likely to have vaginal GBS than women who did not douche.

Chlorhexidine Douching

The most commonly researched substance for vaginal douching for GBS is chlorhexidine; an antibacterial disinfectant. This is used for hand-washing and skin cleansing in many hospitals and is also an ingredient in many medical preparations, including mouthwashes, *Hibiscrub* and *Hibiclens*. Because its effect is transient (which means that, while it may temporarily remove bacteria from an area of the body, once it has worn off they will start to return again), most of the research has centred on looking at whether it can remove GBS bacteria during labour.

A Cochrane review of the use of vaginal chlorhexidine during labour to prevent early-onset GBS disease found five relevant studies including approximately 2190 babies (Stade, et al., 2004). The results were very similar to the results of the review of antibiotics for reducing GBS: the quality of the studies was poor, chlorhexidine use did reduce GBS colonisation in babies but was not associated with a reduction in mortality or other outcomes. For these reasons, the reviewers did not support the use of vaginal disinfection with chlorhexidine in labour for preventing early onset GBS disease, although some women choose to use this treatment as an alternative to intravenous antibiotics (Ross, 2007). Anecdotally, chlorhexidine douching is sometimes combined with douching with other solutions (such as vinegar) and/or live yogurt (to replace 'good' bacteria), but I have not found any useful research on the effectiveness of this practice.

Oral Probiotics

Another theory is that taking oral probiotics or eating live yogurt might help reduce GBS carriage and thus the likelihood of a baby getting GBS disease. Thus far, a very small pilot study including twenty women has taken place in order to test the feasibility of a larger study. The women who took probiotics had lower quantitative GBS colony counts, with the best results in those women who remembered to take the probiotic daily. Having less GBS, of course, is not the same as having no GBS. Although a larger trial would be needed to see if these results were truly significant, the authors of this study felt that further research would be feasible and justified (Hanson, et al., 2014).

Garlic Pessaries

A number of women have tried using garlic pessaries to reduce GBS carriage. Although there is some variation, the most commonly discussed approach is to peel and slightly crush a clove of garlic before inserting it into the vagina overnight. This is done for several nights in a row, and sometimes up until the baby is born. The garlic is removed (or will fall out naturally) each morning. Anecdotally, side effects include itching or a slight burning sensation, which seems to be more likely when the garlic is fresher or when it is heavily crushed before insertion. There has been no research into this, although it has been described in the midwifery literature (Cohain, 2004).

Oral garlic is occasionally mentioned in relation to GBS, along with vitamin C and herbs such as Echinacea, perhaps because they are used by some women as alternatives to antibiotics in other areas of health. However, oral antibiotics have been discarded as ineffective (Gardner, et al., 1979), and it may be that one reason why alternative oral treatments have not has as much attention in this area is that there is a perception that it is more effective to use a preparation locally (that is, in the vagina) in order to reduce GBS carriage in the vagina itself. We do not have enough evidence on this area to know whether such treatments are effective.

Water Birth

Many women want to use water during labour for reasons that have nothing to do with GBS prevention, and I will discuss this topic again in part four, but some people have realised that giving birth in water may in itself be a means of reducing the risk of a baby getting early-onset GBS disease. Although women who are GBS carriers or whose babies are seen to be at risk of getting GBS are usually advised against giving birth in water, Cohain (2010) pointed out that studies of water births show lower rates of GBS disease than are found in the general population. As these water birth studies did not set out to look specifically at GBS, however, we ideally need more research which specifically looks at this issue. The only such study that I could find was carried out by Zanetti-Dällenbach et al. (2007), and included 474 women who used water for labour and/or birth. Of those women, 213 stayed in the water to give birth, while 261 chose to get out before their baby was born. Before they got into the pool, the number of GBS carriers in each group was similar. However, the babies who were born under water were significantly less likely to have GBS than the babies whose mothers laboured in water but gave birth on land. All other outcomes were similar between the groups.

If water birth does reduce the likelihood of a baby being colonised with GBS, there are a number of reasons why this might be the case, and several of these were discussed by Cohain (2010). The water may serve to dilute or wash off GBS bacteria, as evidenced by

Zanetti-Dällenbach et al. (2006), who found GBS in the water that GBS-carrier women had given birth in. Babies born under water may be more likely to stay skin-to-skin with their mothers, which may offer some protection and babies born under water may be less likely to be subject to immediate interventions by comparison to land-born babies. We do need to consider, however, whether this also interferes with the normal colonisation of the baby with healthy bacteria, as with all of the other interventions designed to prevent GBS disease.

Caul birth

Anecdotally, some women and midwives have questioned whether being born in the caul (where the baby's waters do not break until or just after it is being born) is protective against GBS disease. Although there is no systematic research into this (and perhaps will never be), this theory rests on the possibility that the membranes serve as a protective barrier. This is another example of a situation where any reduction in GBS bacteria may also mean a reduction in the bacteria that the baby is meant to pick up during and just after birth.

Arguably, being born in the caul does not really fit as a treatment which may possibly reduce the chance of GBS disease because it is not easily possible to avoid spontaneous rupture of the membranes. It is not a case of being able to say '*I have decided to have my baby born in her caul*' in the same way that one can say, '*I have decided I want to use water during my labour*'. I include it here because some women are asked if they want to have their membranes artificially ruptured by a midwife or doctor, usually as part of the process of induction of labour or in an attempt to speed labour up. (It is not actually an effective way of speeding labour up, and it has potentially undesirable knock-on effects, but that is another book). Women who are concerned about GBS disease, whatever their other choices, may wish to ensure that their membranes (which form the baby's caul) stay intact for as long as possible and avoid other invasive interventions such as vaginal examinations, stretch and sweeps and the use of fetal scalp electrodes.

Future possibilities and ongoing questions

Within medical circles, the main discussion as far as future treatments are concerned is that of a possible vaccine against GBS, not least because even proponents of the current screening and antibiotic treatment regimens are aware that these have *inherent limitations'* (Schrag and Verani, 2013: D20). Oster et al. (2014) recently reported that such a vaccine is in clinical development and that it would theoretically be cost-effective, but whether it would be clinically effective, safe and/or acceptable to women are all important and debatable questions. One of the biggest potential controversies with a vaccine is that it would be offered to all women during pregnancy, as we wouldn't know which women would be at risk of picking up GBS bacteria. On the other hand, concern about antibiotic resistance is growing (Watts, 2014).

Are there other avenues which could usefully be explored? This is purely speculative, but one thing that always strikes me about the research into the majority of the possible treatments for GBS, including antibiotics, chlorhexidine douching and water birth is that, while there is some evidence that all of these might help reduce the chance of a baby being colonised with GBS, we do not know enough about the possible relationship between a reduction in colonisation and a reduction in GBS disease. We do not know the exact mechanism by which GBS disease occurs, for instance, or what other factors may influence this. Some of the researchers who work on this topic have become so focused on eradicating the presence of GBS in the mothers of babies deemed to be at risk that we do not seem to be considering other important things that we do not yet know about this area. Given how much our understanding of bacteria and its importance in our lives has moved on in the past few years, we may be missing the opportunity to reconsider this problem from a different angle, which may lead us to a better solution.

Research into several of the treatments which I have discussed in this part of the book shows that while the treatments appear to reduce GBS carriage, they do not necessarily affect the occurrence of GBS disease in babies. This may be because we have not yet done good enough or large enough research studies. If we did a really good randomised controlled trial, we might show that one or more of these treatments are effective. But it might also be that carrying GBS is only one factor in developing early-onset GBS disease. It might even be that carrying GBS is a necessary starting point for early-onset GBS disease, but that the disease is triggered by something else, which at the moment we don't even know to look for. But as long as there is a possibility that GBS disease has multiple causes, or is caused by something else in the presence of GBS bacteria then the best thing that we can do for our current and future babies is to keep our minds open to other possibilities.

Part Four: Wider issues and making decisions

This final part of the book covers a number of wider issues related to decisions about GBS screening and treatment. The first of these is what happens after the baby is born if there are concerns about GBS, after which I then go on to answer a number of frequently-asked questions about making decisions relating to the issues in this book.

Observing and treating newly born babies

A woman recently asked me why, if doctors are so worried about babies getting GBS, they don't wait for the 'at risk' babies to come out and then give them antibiotics directly. Sometimes that does happen, and I will look at that in this section, but the more usual answer that midwives and doctors give to this question is because (a) research has shown that giving antibiotics to babies can do more harm than good (I will return to this below) and (b) GBS disease can occur so soon after a baby is born that it is thought to be better to get the antibiotics into the baby's system sooner rather than later.

But this may not happen, for one or more reasons. Some women decide not to have antibiotics in labour, for instance, while some plan to have antibiotics but give birth so quickly that there is not time for them to be given. Whatever the situation, where professionals feel that antibiotic coverage has not been adequate, the woman may find that she is offered antibiotics and/or some kind of screening for her baby once it is born.

The screening offered to newborn babies ranges from observation of the baby's condition over a certain period of time to blood tests looking for particular substances such as C-reactive protein (CRP), which indicates the presence of inflammation. Conversations with midwives and doctors around the UK and in other countries has led me to realise that the range of what is offered in these circumstances is incredibly varied, with the following responses being just a few examples:

'If the woman isn't given two doses of antibiotics prior to delivery, baby is recommended to have FBC (full blood count) and CRP at birth, four-hourly observations for 24 hours and then repeat CRP. If the CRP is greater than 7 at birth or greater than 15 at the 24-hour mark, the paediatricians recommend giving intravenous antibiotics to the baby for 48 hours.'

'We don't do specific observations on babies if there has been 2 doses of antibiotics during labour. If less than 2 doses have been given then 4 hourly observations are done for 24 hours. If the baby is stable after 24 hours then s/he can go home.'

'If there are 2 other risk factors such as prolonged rupture of membranes maternal [raised] temperature in labour or prematurity then the babies get IV antibiotics for 48 hours too. I notice a lot of paediatricians use their own discretion here though and put more babies on antibiotics than they should.'

'At our hospital [in Australia], women aren't routinely screened for GBS, unlike in many hospitals. But the paediatricians do a heel prick test on all babies for CRP results at birth instead.'

'In the event of insufficient IV cover (this would be classed as less than 2 doses of antibiotics in labour or the second dose not being on board for at least 1 hour before the infant is born), then neonatal IV antibiotics are usually recommended.'

As I have discussed earlier in the book, antibiotics do carry risks for newborn babies when given directly. We don't know enough about the potential harm to the baby when women are given antibiotics in labour. The use of antibiotics in newly born babies has been associated with a number of unwanted outcomes including asthma, allergies, necrotizing enterocolitis and disseminated fungal infection, some of which can be fatal (Kozyrskyj, et al., 2011, Nash, et al., 2014). They have also been linked with obesity (Ajslev, et al., 2011), psychiatric disorders (Rees, 2014) and an increased chance of the baby being infected with other bacteria which have consequences just as severe as GBS (Edwards , et al., 2002, Bedford Russell and Murch, 2006). In addition, as above, they can prevent the growth of normal, healthy bacteria.

They can also be life-saving for babies who do need them so women and their partners will want to weigh up the risks and the benefits before making the decision that is right for them and their baby. Because of this, and because of the variation in practice in different areas, I would urge any woman who is considering GBS screening or who may have a risk factor to ask about the local guidelines, recommendations and usual practice as early as possible. As I noted in part one, the outcomes of babies who develop GBS disease vary somewhat according to whether a baby was born at full term or preterm. Some women prefer to take a 'wait and see' approach, observing their baby for signs of infection or other problems rather than giving antibiotics just in case.

Some of the midwives and doctors who I talked to shared their discomfort with the way in which women and their partners are sometimes spoken to about their decision to accept antibiotics or not. Because this is seen as a situation in which action must be taken soon after birth, being informed and beginning any conversation about a possible deviation from usual practice ahead of time may be the best approach. AIMS and I know of many women who have chosen to deviate from the usual practice. For instance, one woman told AIMS:

'When I discovered the 'monitoring' at my hospital was likely to involve a doctor or midwife peering into the bassinet every few hours I felt I could do this myself and this confirmed my decision to stay at home. We woke up every couple of hours to take my daughter's temperature, etc.'

It is true that the observation element of monitoring a baby for signs of GBS is mostly a visual examination, and Cantoni et al. (2013) argued from their research that standardised physical examination offered no advantage over standard physical examination plus laboratory tests. The tricky thing about observing babies for infection is that many of the signs of this are signs that can also be seen in normal, healthy newborn babies. They can also appear as subtle changes rather than very obvious problems. For these reasons, and because infection can take hold and become very serious very quickly in newborn babies, a high index of suspicion is usually recommended, which means that it is considered better to check out something that may turn out to be benign than to be unconcerned about a sign that may be an indication of infection, even if it may also be something normal. Some of the signs of infection in babies are listed on the following page, but this should not be considered a substitute for individualised care and advice from a midwife or doctor.

One final point that is worthy of note was raised by an obstetrician:

'Even though we know they aren't 100% effective, we only watch the babies that we decide (arbitrarily based on poor data) to be at increased risk. So does that mean that the ones who got antibiotics but go on to get sick may fall through the cracks?'

Signs of infection in babies

- Baby experiences respiratory distress; seems to be breathing faster than normal, is struggling to breathe, makes grunting or other unusual noises, stops breathing and/or takes long gaps between breaths.

- Baby experiences temperature less than 36°C or more than 38°C, experiences temperature changes (either up or down) or has poor peripheral perfusion (cold or pale hands or feet).

- Baby experiences changes in heart rate or unexpectedly needs resuscitation.

- Baby seems lethargic or floppy, or behaviour or responsiveness seems unusual.

- Baby has feeding difficulties or refuses to feed; baby can't tolerate feed, experiences vomiting and/or has a distended abdomen.

- Baby experiences seizure.

- Baby becomes jaundiced within 24 hours of birth.

- Baby has signs of bleeding, which may manifest as bruises or unusual swelling, especially on the head.

- Other signs of infection in babies include hypoglycaemia (low blood sugar), hypotension (low blood pressure), oxygen desaturation (lowered amount of oxygen being carried in the blood) and metabolic and/or respiratory acidosis. These are not, however, things that can normally be checked without specialised knowledge and/or equipment.

This is a really important point, and one that should be shared with all parents, because in this situation even having every possible test and treatment is no guarantee, and any parent who is concerned about their baby should seek help as quickly as possible, regardless of what testing or treatment they have already received.

GBS and breast milk

Sometimes, women ask whether feeding breast milk to babies is a risk factor for GBS disease. Although there have been a few incidences of late-onset GBS disease in babies whose mothers have then been found to have GBS in their breast milk (Wang, et al., 2007, Jones and Steele, 2012, Filleron, et al., 2014), most women who are carrying GBS do not carry this in their breast milk (Homer, et al., 2014) and, even though some may do, the vast majority of breastfed babies are completely unaffected by GBS in breast milk (Le Doare and Kampmann, 2014). As Berardi et al. (2014) discuss in a recent letter to a paediatric journal, this is a controversial situation for a number of reasons. It is hard to tell whether breast milk samples in some studies have been contaminated, the studies aren't of good quality and there are a number of routes by which GBS can be transmitted, which means we can't be certain from where a baby picked up GBS. Most researchers stress that even rare instances of possible transmission via breast milk are uncertain and vastly outweighed by the positive benefits of breast milk to babies.

Frequently asked questions

This section briefly answers some of the questions which we have been sent and that have either not been directly addressed elsewhere in the book or are so common that we felt they were worth repeating here.

Will I know ahead of time if my baby is deemed to be at risk?

Sometimes yes, for instance if you have previously had a baby with GBS disease or if you have been found to carry GBS on a test, but in many cases, no. Several of the situations discussed in this book which are perceived to constitute risk factors for GBS disease (such as having prolonged rupture of membranes or a raised temperature in labour) will only become apparent once you are near or in labour.

Other than having treatment, are there things I can do to reduce the risk of my baby picking up GBS?

There's not much evidence on this, but avoiding artificial rupture of membranes (where the midwife or doctor breaks your waters) and having as little intervention as possible (including vaginal examinations and stretch and sweeps) might help reduce the chance of your baby getting GBS, and/or reduce the amount of time in which your baby is exposed to GBS. Some midwives believe that it can help to avoid interventions which break the baby's skin, such as the use of a fetal scalp electrode. Having as much skin-to-skin contact between you and your baby as possible after the birth will help colonise the baby with your bacteria, and breastfeeding will confer antibodies to the baby, as well as offering a multitude of other benefits.

If I have a risk factor or a positive GBS test, can I have a water birth?

This will depend a little on where you choose to give birth. If you give birth at home, no-one can stop you using a pool or bath during labour and/or birth. If you give birth in a hospital or birth centre, a pool may not be available or you may be told that you are not able to use it. The answer to this question may also depend on whether or not you have decided to have intravenous antibiotics, although there is no real reason why this should prevent most women using a pool. Some women who have been found to carry GBS have also been told that they are not eligible to use the pool. Unfortunately, there is not much that can be done about either of these situations because institutions do not have an obligation to provide facilities such as pools. It is worth discussing this ahead of time with your midwife, or if using a pool is very important to you, you may wish to consider giving birth at home. Some midwives discourage women from using a birth pool or bath if they have an intravenous cannula in place, but this can easily be covered with a glove (like the midwives themselves wear) and then a bandage around the wrist of the glove in order to keep the cannula as dry as possible. It may be that the midwife asks you to get out of the pool while the antibiotics are given, just in case you have a severe reaction to them.

What do I do if I want GBS screening?

Talk to your midwife and find out what is available locally. You may be able to have this done on the NHS (if you are in the UK) or, if it is not available or you do not consider that the local testing methods are adequate, you may decide you want to have private screening carried out. Usually, midwives and doctors are happy to accept the results of private screening tests, but it may be worth asking whether this will be the case before you pay for screening. Occasionally, women who want to be screened and/or treated for this encounter health professionals who do not seem to understand how important this is to them. If this happens to you, discuss your concerns with your midwife and/or talk to a Supervisor of Midwives.

I want antibiotics in labour. How do I ensure that I get them?

If you have a risk factor or have been found to carry GBS, it is not usually difficult to get antibiotics in labour. In fact, the opposite is true; it can be more difficult to decline antibiotics in labour. But if you are concerned, talk to your midwife and ask to have a plan of care made before you go into labour.

I'm having a hospital birth. Will having antibiotics affect when I go into hospital in labour?

Women who know that they are carrying GBS and who decide ahead of time to have antibiotics when they go into labour are sometimes advised to go to hospital as soon as their labour starts. This is so that there is the maximum possible chance that they will receive two doses of antibiotics before their baby is born. However, there are risks to going into hospital in early labour, including that there is a higher chance of having certain interventions, including pain relief. As discussed elsewhere, antibiotics are not usually given until labour is established, but there is a balance to be struck here between wanting to make sure that labour is established (in order to prevent antibiotics being given unnecessarily) and wanting to ensure that antibiotics are started early enough that two doses will have been given before the baby is born.

Somewhat paradoxically, some of the women who go in early (as they were told to) are sometimes then sent home again by another midwife or doctor without having had antibiotics. This can be immensely frustrating. I know of cases where women who did not want to stay in hospital at that point went in, had a dose of antibiotics, stayed long enough to ensure they were not having an allergic reaction, and then went home again. There are many possible permutations and situations and, overall, the best advice for women who are in this situation is to discuss a plan of care ahead of time with their midwife or doctor.

I am worried that being screened for GBS will affect my planned home / birth centre birth?

You can, unfortunately, be denied entrance to a birth centre or midwifery-led unit, but no-one can deny you the right to give birth in your own home and, in the UK, midwives have a duty of care to attend you. You can decline screening if you do not want this and/ or are concerned that this will affect your care. Despite having these rights, having a risk factor for GBS and/or being found to be positive for GBS can mean you come under pressure. You could talk to your midwife and find out what the situation would be locally. If you do not get the support you need, you could talk to a Supervisor of Midwives or contact AIMS.

I don't want to be screened for GBS. How can I make sure this doesn't happen?

Screening is not compulsory and you can decline any screening test that you do not want to have. However, it is important to remember that GBS screening is not always presented as such in the UK, and that GBS may be found anytime that a vaginal or perianal swab or urine sample is tested. (This does not apply to urine tests that are done during antenatal visits; only when a urine sample is collected in a pot and sent to a laboratory). If you are offered such a test, you can ask what it is for, why the midwife or doctor thinks it is necessary and what will happen when the results come back. If you are concerned about the implications of such testing for your options in labour, you should discuss this with the midwife or doctor before agreeing to the test. You always have the right to decline having a test, to ask for a second opinion, or to speak to a Supervisor of Midwives or Consultant Midwife (if available) for further support.

My GBS test was positive or I have a risk factor but I don't want antibiotics in labour?

You do not have to consent to anything that you do not want to have. Your midwife or doctor may be (or feel) obliged to offer antibiotics and to ensure that you have full information about what is being suggested, but it is your body and your choice.

Can I have a home birth if I have a risk factor for GBS?

No test result or risk factor can prevent you from having a home birth. You are not obliged to go to hospital or anywhere else to give birth, and you are not obliged to consent to anything that you do not want to consent to. Depending on where you live and on the quality of the local service, you may have no problem, or you may find that pressure is put upon you to go into hospital, or that you are told that a midwife may not be able to attend your birth. If you are in the UK, AIMS' book *Am I Allowed?* contains more information on this. Women in other countries may be able to find out more through home birth groups, midwives or organisations in their country. If you want to have intravenous antibiotics, however, you may find that you are told that it is not possible to have these at home. Refer to pages 95-98 for more on this.

Can I get alternative treatments for GBS on the NHS?

As things currently stand, it is unusual to get support for or information about alternative remedies from midwives or doctors who work in the NHS or other systems of maternity care. This is because they have to follow guidance and these remedies are not officially recommended. You will find information elsewhere (including on the internet) but please remember that such information is of hugely variable quality and that so-called 'natural' remedies can also have unwanted side effects.

I can't get the information I need from my midwife or doctor

Every UK hospital always has a Supervisor of Midwives on call, and you can call the hospital switchboard and ask to speak to her or him. If your local hospital or Trust has one, you could also try contacting a Consultant Midwife.

What sort of plan of care might be negotiated by someone who doesn't want antibiotics?

If a woman who is known to be GBS positive or have risk factors wishes to decline antibiotics, then it is fairly common for a Supervisor of Midwives to get involved, ideally with involvement from the woman's named midwife as well. The Supervisor of Midwives will want to ensure that the woman has been given appropriate information and they will develop a plan of care together. Women who have taken this approach in recent years have found that the most common plan of care is that the baby will be observed every four hours in the hospital for the first 24 hours, with further discussion about antibiotics for the baby if she or he shows signs of infection. Women who have wanted a home birth and no antibiotics have negotiated a plan whereby they do this and a midwife visits a couple of times within the first 24 hours and closely observes the baby for signs of infection. In this situation, the women observe their baby in between these visits, following good instruction from the midwife, with signs of infection and details of when to call for help clearly written down. Remember that you do not have to agree to anything that you do not want to.

I declined antibiotics but have now been told that my baby must have them – can I decline?

This can be a tricky situation, because women and their partners can find themselves under a great deal of pressure to have antibiotics given to their baby, and some women have even been threatened with legal action and/or being reported to Social Services. The important thing to understand in this situation is that, while all decisions rest with the woman while the baby is unborn, a newborn baby is a person in their own right who has rights of their own. Doctors who look after newborn babies have a legal duty of care to those babies, and if they feel that parents are recklessly compromising a baby's health, they do have a degree of legal power. As the Birthrights fact sheet on consent explains:

> "Consent for any medical treatment or procedure, including the administration of a drug, must be sought from a person with 'parental responsibility' for the baby. This always includes the baby's mother, but the baby's father has parental responsibility only if certain criteria are met. You can find a summary of parental responsibility on the NHS Choices website.

If parents refuse treatment for their child, healthcare professionals should respect their decision. In some circumstances, including if parents disagree about treatment, healthcare professionals may approach the High Court for an order declaring that treatment is in a child's best interests and should be carried out." (Birthrights, 2013: 4)

Some people feel that the key is to ensure that you do not give the doctor or other staff any reason to think that you are being reckless or unreasonable. It can help to stay calm, be clear about your concerns and engage in a two-way conversation, thus demonstrating that you are open to discussion and respectful of the staff's expertise (even if this is not how you feel). You may wish to explain your understanding that GBS disease is rare and that you are concerned about the long-term risks of antibiotics to your baby's health, which are relatively unknown.

'We explained [to the] neonatologist that we were concerned about possible side effects, later antibiotic resistance, gut problems and other negative consequences of antibiotics. I think it helped to use the medical terms, and definitely it helped to be calm and let them know that we really understood the risks of GBS. We said we were happy for our baby to be observed and that we wouldn't oppose antibiotics if there were actual signs of infection, and I offered to sign a page in my notes where we wrote this plan down, but that I didn't want him to have antibiotics just in case.'

You could try contacting a Supervisor of Midwives and/or a Consultant Midwife for support, especially if they have been helpful to you in the past, but their role is a little different in this situation. You are more likely to encounter the 'safeguarding' midwife, whose role is more about the protection of babies. AIMS is always happy to support women who experience difficulties in this kind of situation, and details of how to contact both AIMS and Birthrights are given in the resources section at the back of this book.

In conclusion

Once this book is published, I am almost certain that it will be criticised in some circles because I haven't urged women to take every test possible and agree to intravenous antibiotics during labour. However, I hope I haven't made my reader think that GBS is something to dismiss, or that having antibiotics is always inadvisable. As is so often the case in decisions relating to pregnancy and birth, the evidence is unclear and often lacking, the options can weigh heavily and no decision comes with a guarantee. GBS can cause a life-threatening and sometimes fatal disease, but the vast majority of women who carry it won't be affected, and neither will their babies. Accepting the interventions that are on offer does not offer a guarantee, though it may limit a woman's options and confer other risks. But the fact that we can't always prevent GBS disease and that our efforts to prevent GBS disease can cause other problems doesn't make it less of a life-threatening disease to those few babies who get it.

Quite understandably, some of those people whose babies have been lost to GBS disease are among those seeking to inform other women and families about the issue, and are some of the strongest proponents of screening and antibiotic treatment. If you want to read published accounts of women's experiences of losing babies to GBS disease, you could look at the book 'Mourning Sarah: a case for testing group B strep' (Huttlinger Vigour, 2009) or the articles by Bodard-Williams

(2013) or the anonymous mother (Anon, 2001) who shared her story in an AIMS Journal.

AIMS and I know from the women who contact us that the campaigns for GBS awareness are seen as incredibly positive by some people and as incredibly disempowering by others:

> 'My 'journey' into maternity rights started when a huge yellow sticker (which made me feel a pariah at all appointments) was stuck onto my red book (maternity notes) without my consent. This was provided by the GBSS group and said "Give Antibiotics when in labour". When I questioned it, I was told I had no choice…'

> 'I will always support the GBS campaign as I might have lost my baby if not for their information.'

> 'GBS is shrouded in a lot of confusion and misunderstanding - there are a lot of frightening sounding statistics used on sites that are clearly very biased towards hospital births with antibiotics for all.'

> 'Women don't realise that they have choices and options beyond what they are presented with by NHS staff. For example, I was told by a nice and well-meaning yet not knowledgeable on the subject community midwife that being GBS positive meant that I "wouldn't get my lovely homebirth". I ended up after a lot of research opting for the antibiotics in early labour and then going home again.'

Ultimately, it is up to you whether you have screening for GBS, it is up to you whether you have intravenous antibiotics in labour or not and it is up to you whether or not you want your healthy baby to have antibiotics 'just in case'. Whatever it is that you decide I hope this book has helped explain the issues relating to GBS and helped you in making the decision that is right for you. If you need further information or support, you will find details of organisations that may be able to help you on page 144. If you would like to support other women, or help to ensure that AIMS can keep funding books like this one, please consider becoming a member and supporting the organisation in its work. You can find details of how to join on page 151.

References

AAP, 1992. American Academy of Pediatrics Committee on Infectious Diseases and Committee on Fetus and Newborn. Guidelines for prevention of group B streptococcal infection by chemoprophylaxis. *Pediatrics,* Volume 90, pp. 775-8.

Abdelazim, I. A., 2013. Intrapartum polymerase chain reaction for detection of group B streptococcus colonisation. *Australian and New Zealand Journal of Obstetrics and Gynaecology,* 53(3), pp. 236-242.

ACOG, 1992. Committee on Technical Bulletins of the American College of Obstetricians and Gynecologists Group B streptococcal infections in pregnancy, *ACOG Technical Bulletin* 170.

Adriaenssens, N., Coenen, S., Versporten, A., et al., 2011. European Surveillance of Antimicrobial Consumption (ESAC): outpatient antibiotic use in Europe (1997–2009). *J Antimicrob Chemother,* 66(Suppl 6), p. vi3–12.

Ajslev, T. A., Andersen, C. S., Gamborg, M., et al. 2011. Childhood overweight after establishment of the gut microbiota: the role of delivery mode, pre-pregnancy weight and early administration of antibiotics. *Int J Obes (Lond) ,* Volume 35, p. 522–9.

Alfirevic, Z., Gyte, G. M. & Dou, L., 2010. Different classes of antibiotics given to women routinely for preventing infection at caesarean section, *Cochrane Database of Systematic Reviews* 2010, Issue 10.

Ambrose, N. S., Johnson, M., Burdon, D. W., et al., 1985. The influence of single dose intravenous antibiotics on faecal flora and emergence of Clostridium difficile. *J. Antimicrob. Chemother.,* 15(3), pp. 319-326.

Andersen, J. T., Petersen, M., Jimenez-Solem, E., et al., 2013. Clarithromycin in early pregnancy and the risk of miscarriage and malformation: a register based nationwide cohort study. *PLoS ONE* .

Anon, 2001. Caroline's Story. *AIMS Journal,* 13(3), pp. 15-17.

Ashkenazi-Hoffnung, L., Melamed, N. & Ben-Haroush, A., 2011. The Association of Intrapartum Antibiotic Exposure With the Incidence and Antibiotic Resistance of Infantile Late-Onset Serious Bacterial Infections. *Clin Pediatric,* 50(9), pp. 827-833.

Baker, C. J. & Barrett, F. F., 1973. Transmission of group B streptococci among parturient women and their neonates. *Journal of Pediatrics,* Volume 83, pp. 919-25.

Barber, E. L., Zhao, G., Buhimschi, I. A., et al., 2008. Duration of intrapartum prophylaxis and concentration of penicillin G in fetal serum at delivery. *Obstetrics and Gynecology,* 112(2), pp. 265-270.

Barcaite, E., Bartusevicius, A., Tameliene, R., et al., 2008. Prevalence of maternal group B streptococcal colonisation in European countries. *Acta Obstetricia et Gynecologica Scandinavica,* 87(3), pp. 260-271.

Barcaite, E., Bartusevicius, A. & Tameliene, R., et al., 2012. Group B streptococcus and Escherichia coli colonization in pregnant women and neonates in Lithuania. *Int J Gynecology and Obstetrics,* 117(1), pp. 69-73.

Bedford Russell, A. R. & Murch, S., 2006. Could peripartum antibiotics have delayed health consequences for the infant? *BJOG,* 113(7), pp. 758-765.

Berardi A, D. F. G., G. S., et al., 2011. Universal antenatal screening for group B streptococcus in Emilia-Romagna. *J Med Screening,* 18(2), pp. 60-64.

Berardi, A., Rossi, C., Guidotti, I., et al., 2014. Group B streptococci in milk and neonatal colonisation. *Arch Dis Childhood,* 99(4), p. 395.

Berthier, A., Senthiles, L., Hamou, L., et al., 2007. Antibiotics at term. Questions about five allergic accidents. *Gynécologie, Obstétrique & Fertilité,* Volume 35, p. 464–72.

Birthrights, 2013. *Consenting to treatment.* [Online] Available at: http://www.birthrights.org.uk/library/factsheets/ Consenting-to-Treatment.pdf

Blaser, M., 2011. Antibiotic overuse: Stop the killing of beneficial bacteria. *Nature,* Volume 476, p. 393–394.

Bodard-Williams, C., 2013. Group B strep infection: a mother's perspective. *The Practising Midwife,* 16(2), pp. 17-19.

Broe, A., Pottegård, A., Lamont, R. F., et al., 2014. Increasing use of antibiotics in pregnancy during the period 2000–2010: prevalence, timing, category, and demographics. *BJOG,* 121(8), pp. 988-96.

Cantoni, L., Ronfani, L., Da Riol, R., et al., 2013. Physical examination instead of laboratory tests for most infants born to mothers colonized with group B Streptococcus: support for the centers for Disease Control and Prevention's 2010 recommendations. *J Pediat,* 163(2), pp. 568-573.e1.

Carstensen, H., Christensen, K. K., Grennert, L., et al., 1988. Early-onset neonatal group B streptococcal septicaemia in siblings. *J Infect,* 17(3), pp. 201-4.

CDC, see Centers for Disease Control and Prevention

Centers for Disease Control and Prevention, 2005. Early-onset and late-onset neonatal group B streptococcal disease-United States, 1996-2004. *Morbidity and Mortality Weekly Report,* 54(47), pp. 1205-8.

Centers for Disease Control and Prevention, 2007. Perinatal group B streptococcal disease after universal screening recommendations-United States, 2003-2005. *Morbidity and Mortality Weekly Report,* Volume 56, pp. 701-5.

Centers for Disease Control and Prevention, 2010. *Prevention of perinatal group B streptococcal disease: revised guidelines from CDC, 2010. Morbidity and Mortality Weekly Report 2010;* 59(RR-10), pp. 1-36.

Chan, G., Modak, J., Mahmud, A., et al., 2013. Maternal and neonatal colonization in Bangladesh: prevalences, etiologies and risk factors. *J Perinatol,* 33(12), pp. 971-976.

Chan, W. S. W. et al., 2014. Rapid identification of group B streptococcus carriage by PCR to assist in the management of women with prelabour rupture of membranes in term pregnancy. *ANZJOG,* 54(2), pp. 138-145.

Chaudhuri, K., Gonzales, J., Jesurun, C. A., et al., 2008. Anaphylactic shock in pregnancy: a case study and review of the literature. *Int J Obstet Anesth,* Volume 17, p. 350–7.

Christensen, K. K., Christensen, P., Dahlander, K., et al., 1983. The significance of group B streptococci in neonatal pneumonia. *Europ J Pediatrics,* Issue 140, pp. 118-22.

Cohain, J. S., 2004. GBS, pregnancy and garlic: be a part of the solution. *Midwifery Today,* Volume 72, pp. 24-25.

Cohain, J. S., 2010. Newborn group B strep infection. Top 10 reasons not to culture at 36 weeks. *Midwifery Today,* Volume 94, p. 15.

Colbourn, T. & Gilbert, R., 2007. An overview of the natural history of early onset group B streptococcal disease in the UK. *Early Human Development,* 83(3), pp. 149-156.

Collado, M. C., Cernada, M., Baüerl, C., et al., 2012. Microbial ecology and host-microbiota interactions during early life stages. *Gut Microbes,* 3(4), p. 352–365.

Dadvand, P., Basagana, X., Figueras, F., et al., 2011. Climate and group B streptococci colonisation during pregnancy: present implications and future concerns. *BJOG,* 118(11), pp. 1396-1400.

Daniels, J., Gray, J., Pattison, H., et al., 2009. Rapid testing for group B streptococcus during labour: a test accuracy study with evaluation of acceptability and cost-effectiveness. *Health Tech Assmt,* 13(42), p. 178.

de Steenwinkel, F., Tak, H. & Muller, A., et al., 2008. Low carriage rate of group B streptococcus in pregnant women in Maputo, Mozambique. *Trop Med Int Health,* 13(3), pp. 427-429.

Dillon, H. C., Khare, S. & Gray, B. M., 1987. Group B streptococcal carriage and disease: a 6-year prospective study. *J Pediat,* Volume 110, pp. 31-6.

Dinsmoor, M. J., Viloria, R., Leif, L., et al., 2005. Use of intrapartum antibiotics and the incidence of postnatal maternal and neonatal yeast infections. *O&G,* Volume 106, pp. 19-22.

Dunn, A. B., Blomquist, J. & Khouzami, V., 1999. Anaphylaxis in labor secondary to prophylaxis against group B streptococcus: a case report. *J Repro Med,* 44(4), pp. 381-384.

Eastwood, K. A., Craig, S., Sidhu, H., et al., 2014. Prevention of early-onset Group B Streptococcal disease – the Northern Ireland experience. *BJOG.* DOI: 10.1111/1471-0528.12841

Edwards, R. K., Clark, P., Sistrom, C. L., et al., 2002. Intrapartum antibiotic prophylaxis 1: Relative effects of recommended antibiotics on gram-negative pathogens. *O&G,* Volume 100, pp. 534-9.

El Helali, N., Giovangrandi, Y., Guyot, K., et al., 2012. Cost and effectiveness of intrapartum group B streptococcus polymerase chain reaction screening for term deliveries. *O&G,* 119(4), pp. 822-829.

Fairlie, T., Zell, E. R. & Schrag, S., 2013. Effectiveness of intrapartum antibiotic prophylaxis for prevention of early-onset group B streptococcal disease. *Obstet Gynecol,* Volume 121, p. 570–577.

Faro, J. P., Bishop, K., Riddle, G., et al., 2013. Accuracy of an accelerated, culture-based assay for detection of group B streptococcus. *Infect Dis in O&G,* 2013:367935. DOI: 10.1155/2013/367935.

Filleron, A., Lombard, F., Jacquot, A., et al., 2014. Group B streptococci in milk and late neonatal infections: an analysis of cases in the literature. *Arch Dis Childhood,* Fet Neonat Ed 99(1), pp. F41-F47.

Florindo, C., Damiao, V., Lima, J., et al., 2014. Accuracy of prenatal culture in predicting intrapartum group B streptococcus colonization status. *J Mat-Fetal Neonat Med,* 27(6), pp. 640-642.

Gardner, S. E., Yow, M. D., Leeds, L. J., et al., 1979. Failure of penicillin to eradicate group B streptococcal colonization in the pregnant woman. A couple study. *Am J Obstet Gynecol ,* Volume 135, p. 1062–5.

Garland, S. M., 1991. Early onset neonatal group B streptococcus (GBS) infection: associated obstetric risk factors. *ANZJOG,* Volume 10, pp. 801-8.

Garland, S. M. & Kelly, N., 1995. A study of Group B Streptococcus in Brisbane; the epidemiology, detection by PCR assay and serovar prevalence. *Med J Austral,* Volume 162, pp. 413-417.

Gilbert, R., 2014. Immediate delivery for group B streptococci-colonised women with preterm premature rupture of membranes. Don't forget the antibiotics. *BJOG.* DOI: 10.1111/1471-0528.12940

Glasgow, T. S., Speakman, M., Firth, S., et al., 2007. Clinical and economic outcomes for term infants associated with increasing administration of antibiotics to their mothers. *Paed Perinat Epid,* 21(4), pp. 338-346.

Grimwood, K., Stone, P. R., Gosling, I. A., et al., 2002. Late antenatal carriage of group B Streptococcus by New Zealand women. *ANZJOG,* 42(2), pp. 182-86.

Grönlund, M. M., Lehtonen, O. P., Eerola, E., et al., 1999. Fecal microflora in healthy infants born by different methods of delivery: permanent changes in intestinal flora after cesarean delivery. *J Pediatr Gastroenterol Nutr,* 28(1), pp. 19-25.

Håkansson, S. & Källén, K., 2006. Impact and risk factors for early-onset group B streptococcal morbidity: analysis of a national, population-based cohort in Sweden 1997-2001. *BJOG,* Volume 113, pp. 1452-8.

Håkansson, S., Källén, K., Bullarbo, M., et al., 2014. Real-time PCR-assay in the delivery suite for determination of group B streptococcal colonization in a setting with risk-based antibiotic prophylaxis. *J Mat-Fetal Neonat Med,* 27(4), pp. 328-332.

Hanson, L., VandeVusse, L., Duster, M., et al., 2014. Feasibility of Oral Prenatal Probiotics against Maternal Group B Streptococcus Vaginal and Rectal Colonization. *JOGNN,* 43(3), pp. 294-304.

Heath, P.T., Balfour, G., Weisner, A. M., et al., 2004. PHLS Group B Streptococcus Working Group. Group B streptococcal disease in UK and Irish infants younger than 90 days. *Lancet*, Volume 363, p. 292–4.

Homer, S. E., Scarf, V., Catling, C., et al., 2014. Culture-based versus risk-based screening for the prevention of group B streptococcal disease in newborns: A review of national guidelines. *Women and Birth,* Volume 27, pp. 46-51.

Hong, J., Choi, C., Park, K., et al., 2010. Genital group B streptococcus carrier rate and serotype distribution in Korean pregnant women: implications for group B streptococcal disease in Korean neonates. *J Perinat Med,* 38(4), pp. 373-377.

Huttlinger Vigour, T., 2009. *Mourning Sarah: a case for testing group B strep.* Abingdon: Radcliffe Publishing.

Jamie, W. E., Edwards, R. K. & Duff, P., 2004. Vaginal-perianal compared with vaginal-rectal cultures for identification of group B streptococci. *Obstet Gynecol,* 104(5 Pt 1), pp. 1058-1061.

Jao, M. S., Cheng, P. J., Shaw, S. W., et al., 2006. Anaphylaxis to cefazolin during labor secondary to prophylaxis for group B Streptococcus: a case report. *J Repro Med,* 51(8), pp. 655-8.

Joachim, A., Matee, M. I., Massawe, F. A., et al., 2009. Maternal and neonatal colonisation of group B streptococcus at Muhimbili National Hospital in Dar es Salaam, Tanzania: prevalence, risk factors and antimicrobial resistance. *BMC Public Health,* Volume 9, p. 437.

Jones, S. M. & Steele, R. W., 2012. Recurrent group B streptococcal bacteremia. *Clin Pediatrics,* 51(9), pp. 884-887.

Kaambwa, B., Bryan, S., Gray, J., et al., 2010. Cost-effectiveness of rapid tests and other existing strategies for screening and management of early-onset group B streptococcus during labour. *BJOG,* 117(13), pp. 1616-1627.

Kenyon, S., Taylor, D. J. & Tarnow-Mordi, W., 2001a. Broad spectrum antibiotics for preterm, prelabour rupture of fetal membranes: the ORACLE I randomised trial. *Lancet,* Volume 357, p. 979–88.

Kenyon, S. L., Taylor, D. J. & Tarnow-Mordi, W., 2001b. Broad-spectrum antibiotics for spontaneous preterm labour: the ORACLE II randomised trial. *Lancet,* 357(9261), pp. 989-94.

Khan, R., Anastasakis, E. & Kadir, R., 2008. Anaphylactic reaction to ceftriaxone in labour. An emerging complication. *J Obs Gyn,* 28(7), pp. 751-753.

Knight, K. M., Thornburg, L. L., McNanley, A. R., et al., 2012. The effect of intrapartum clindamycin on vaginal group B streptococcus colony counts. *J Mat-Fet Neonat Med* 25(6):747-749.

Knudtson E.J., L. L., S. V., et al., 2010. The effect of digital cervical examination on group B streptococcal culture. *AJOG,* 202(1), pp. 58.e1-58.e4.

Kovavisarach, E., Jarupisarnlert, P. & Kanjanaharuetai, S. J., 2008. The accuracy of late antenatal screening cultures in predicting intrapartum group B streptococcal colonization. *Med Assoc Thai,* 291(12), pp. 1796-800.

Kozyrskyj, A. L., Bahreinian, S. & Azad, M. B., 2011. Early life exposures: impact on asthma and allergic disease. *Curr Opin Allergy Clin Immunol,* Volume 11, p. 400–6.

Kunze M, Z. A., F. K., et al., 2011. Colonization, serotypes and transmission rates of group B streptococci in pregnant women and their infants born at a single University Center in Germany. *J Perinat Med*, 39(4), pp. 417-422.

Larsen, J. W. & Sever, J. L., 2008. Group B Streptococcus and pregnancy: a review. *Am J Obstet Gynecol*, 198(4), pp. 440-50.

Le Doare, K. & Kampmann, B., 2014. Breast milk and Group B streptococcal infection: Vector of transmission or vehicle for protection? *Vaccine*, 32(26), pp. 3128-32.

Ledger, W. J., 2006. Prophylactic antibiotics in obstetrics–gynecology: a current asset, a future liability? *Expert Review of Anti-infective Therapy*, 4(6), pp. 957-964.

Lee, B., Song, Y., Kim, M., et al., 2010. Epidemiology of group B streptococcus in Korean pregnant women. *Epidemiology and Infection*, 138(2), pp. 292-298.

MacDonald, C., McLachlan, R., Handorf, S. & Green, J., 2010. Group B Streptococcus: The impact of risk and prophylaxis on midwives and women in the childbirth experience. *Birthspirit Midwifery Journal*, Volume 6, pp. 47-54.

Mavenyengwa, R. T., Afset, J. E., Schei, B., et al., 2010. Group B Streptococcus colonization during pregnancy and maternal-fetal transmission in Zimbabwe. *Acta Obst et Gyn Scand*, 89(2), pp. 250-255.

McNanley, A. R., Glantz, C., Hardy, D. J. et al., 2007. The effect of intrapartum penicillin on vaginal group B streptococcus colony counts. *AJOG*, 197(6), pp. 583-5.e1-4.

Money, D., Dobson, S., Cole, L., et al., 2008. An evaluation of a rapid real time polymerase chain reaction assay for detection of group B streptococcus as part of a neonatal group B streptococcus prevention strategy. *JOGC*, 30(9), pp. 770-775.

Morinis, J., Shah, J., Murthy, P., et al., 2011. Horizontal transmission of group B streptococcus in a neonatal intensive care unit. *Paediatrics and Child Health*, 16(6), pp. 329-330.

Mueller, M., Henle, A., Droz, S., et al., 2014. Intrapartum detection of Group B streptococci colonization by rapid PCR-test on labor ward. *Euro J of Obs Gyn Repro Biol*, Volume 176, pp. 137-141.

Nash, C., Simmons, E., Bhagat, P., et al., 2014. Antimicrobial stewardship in the NICU: lessons we've learned. *NeoReviews*, 15(4), pp. e116-e122.

National Institute for Health and Clinical Excellence, 2008a. *Antenatal Care*, NICE Clinical Guideline No. 62, London: NICE.

National Institute for Health and Clinical Excellence, 2008b. *Induction of labour*, NICE Clinical Guideline No. 70, London: NICE.

National Institute for Health and Clinical Excellence, 2011. *Caesarean Section*, NICE Clinical Guideline No. 132, London: NICE.

National Institute for Health and Clinical Excellence, 2012. *Antibiotics for early-onset neonatal infection: Antibiotics for the prevention and treatment of early-onset neonatal infection*, NICE Clinical Guideline No. 149, London: NICE.

National Institute for Health and Clinical Excellence, 2013. Induction of labour Evidence Update July 2013. *A summary of selected new evidence relevant to NICE clinical guideline 70 'Induction of labour' (2008) Evidence Update 44*, London: NICE.

Neu, J., 2007. Perinatal and neonatal manipulation of the intestinal microbiome: a note of caution. *Nutr Rev*, Volume 65, p. 282–5.

Nguyen, T. M., Gauthier, D. W., M. T., et al., 1998. Detection of group B streptococcus: comparison of an optical immunoassay with direct plating and broth-enhanced culture methods. *J Matern Fetal Med*, 7(4), pp. 172-6.

NHS Choices, 2014. *Side effects of antibiotics*. [Online] Available at: www.nhs.uk/Conditions/Antibiotics-penicillins/Pages/Side-effects.aspx

NICE, see National Institute for Health and Clinical Excellence

Oddie, S. & Embleton, N. D., 2002. Risk factors for early onset neonatal group B streptococcal sepsis: case–control study. *BMJ*, Volume 325, p. 308.

Ohlsson, A. & Shah, V., 2014. Intrapartum antibiotics for known maternal Group B streptococcal colonization. (Cochrane Review). (Last assessed as up-to-date: 11 March 2014). *Cochrane Database of Systematic Reviews 2014*, Issue 6. Art. No.: CD007467. DOI: 10.1002/14651858.CD007467.pub4.

Onderdonk, A. B., Delaney, M. L., Hinkson, P. L., DuBois, A. M., et al., 1992. Quantitative and qualitative effects of douche preparations on vaginal microflora. *Obstet Gynecol*, Volume 80, pp. 333-338.

Onwuchuruba, C. N., Towers, C. V., Howard, B.C., et al., 2014. Transplacental passage of vancomycin from mother to neonate. AJOG, 210(4), pp. 352-354.

Oster, G., Edelsberg, J. & Hennegan, K., 2002. Prevention of group B streptococcal disease in the first 3 months of life: Would routine maternal immunization during pregnancy be cost-effective? Vaccine, 32(37), pp. 4778-85.

Pelaez, L. M., Gelber, S. E., Fox, N. S., et al., 2009. Inappropriate use of vancomycin for preventing perinatal group B streptococcal (GBS) disease in laboring patients. J Perinat Med, 37(5), pp. 487-489.

Poncelet-Jasserand, E., Forges, F., Varlet, M. N., et al., 2013. Reduction of the use of antimicrobial drugs following the rapid detection of Streptococcus agalactiae in the vagina at delivery by real-time PCR assay. BJOG, 120(9), pp. 1098-1109.

RCOG, see Royal College of Obstetricians and Gynaecologists

Rees, J. C., 2014. Obsessive-compulsive disorder and gut microbiota dysregulation. Med Hypotheses, 82(2), pp. 163-6.

Ross, S., 2007. Chlorhexidine as an alternative treatment for prevention of group B streptococcal disease. Midwifery Today, Volume 82, pp. 42-43, 68.

Royal College of Obstetricians and Gynaecologists, 2003. Prevention of early onset neonatal group B streptococcal disease. Green top guideline No 36. London: RCOG.

Royal College of Obstetricians and Gynaecologists, 2012. Prevention of early onset neonatal group B streptococcal disease, Green top guideline No 36. London: RCOG. http://www.rcog.org.uk/files/rcog-corp/GTG36_GBS.pdf

Royal College of Obstetricians and Gynaecologists, 2013. *Group B streptococcus (GBS) infection in newborn babies. Patient Information leaflet,* http://www.rcog.org.uk/files/rcog-corp/PI_GroupB_ streptococcus_%28GBS%29_infection_in_newborn_babies.pdf

Sakru, N., Inceboz, T., Inceboz, U., et al., 2006. Does vaginal douching affect the risk of vaginal infections in pregnant women? *Saudi Med J,* 27(2), pp. 215-218.

Schrag, S. J., et al., 2002. A population-based comparison of strategies to prevent early-onset group B streptococcal disease in neonates. *NEJM,* Volume 347, pp. 233-9.

Schrag, S. J. & Verani, J. R., 2013. Intrapartum antibiotic prophylaxis for the prevention of perinatal group B streptococcal disease: experience in the United States and implications for a potential group B streptococcal vaccine. *Vaccine,* 31(Suppl 4), pp. D20-6.

Schuchat, A., 1999. Group B streptococcus. *Lancet,* 353(9146), pp. 51-56.

Seale, J. & Millar, M., 2014. Perinatal vertical transmission of antibiotic-resistant bacteria: a systematic review and proposed research strategy. *BJOG,* 121(8), pp. 923-8.

Seoud M, N. A., Z. P., et al., 2010. Prenatal and neonatal Group B Streptococcus screening and serotyping in Lebanon: incidence and implications. *Acta Obst Gyn Scand,* 89(3), pp. 399-403.

Shore, E. M. & Yudin, M. H., 2012. Choice of antibiotic for group B streptococcus in women in labour based on antibiotic sensitivity testing. *JOGC,* 34(3), pp. 230-235.

Singleton, M. L., 2007. Group B strep prophylaxis: what are we creating? *Midwifery Today,* Volume 81, pp. 18-20.

Stade, B., Shah, V. & Ohlsson, A., 2004. *Vaginal chlorhexidine during labour to prevent early-onset neonatal group B streptococcal infection. The Cochrane Database of Systematic Reviews*, Issue 1, 2004.

Stapleton, R. D., Kahn, J. M., Evans, L. E., et al., 2005. Risk factors for group B streptococcal genitourinary tract colonization in pregnant women. *O&G*, 106(6), pp. 1246-1252.

Stokholm, J., Schjørring, S., Eskildsen, C. E., et al., 2013. Antibiotic use during pregnancy alters the commensal vaginal microbiota. *Clin Microbiol Infect*, 20(7), pp. 629-35.

Stoll, B. J., et al., 2011. Early onset neonatal sepsis: the burden of Group B Streptococcal and E. coli disease continues. *Pediatrics*, 127(5), pp. 817-26.

Tajik, P., van der Ham, D., Zafarmand, M., et al., 2014. Using vaginal Group B Streptococcus colonisation in women with preterm premature rupture of membranes to guide the decision for immediate delivery: a secondary analysis of the PPROMEXIL trials. *BJOG*, DOI: 10.1111/1471-0528.12889.

The CAESAR study collaborative group, 2010. Caesarean section surgical techniques: a randomised factorial trial (CAESAR). *BJOG*, Volume 117, p. 1366–1376.

Towers, C. V., Howard, B. C. & Onwuchuruba, C. N., 2014. Vancomycin dosage for group B streptococcus prophylaxis - response. *AJOG*, DOI: http://dx.doi.org/10.1016/j.ajog.2014.06.040.

Trappe, K. L., Shaffer, L. E. & Stempel, L. E., 2011. Vaginal-perianal compared with vaginal-rectal cultures for detecting group B streptococci during pregnancy. *O&G*, 118(2 part 1), pp. 313-317.

Tse, H., Wong, S. C. Y. & Sridhar, S., 2014. Vancomycin dosage for group B streptococcus prophylaxis. *AJOG.* DOI: http://dx.doi.org/10.1016/j.ajog.2014.06.040.

Turnbaugh, P. J., Ley, R. E., Hamady, M., et al., 2007. The human microbiome project. *Nature,* Volume 449, p. 804–10.

Turrentine, M.A., Greisinger, A.J., Brown, K.S., et al., 2013. Duration of intrapartum antibiotics for group B streptococcus on the diagnosis of clinical neonatal sepsis. *Infect Dis Obstet Gynecol,* 2013:525878. DOI: 10.1155/2013/525878.

Turrentine, M., 2014. Intrapartum antibiotic prophylaxis for Group B Streptococcus: has the time come to wait more than 4 hours? *AJOG,* 211(1), pp. 15-17.

UK National Screening Committee, 2008. *Group B Streptococcus: The UK NSC policy on Group B Streptococcus screening in pregnancy,* London: NSC. http://www.screening.nhs.uk/groupbstreptococcus

Valkenburg-van den Berg, A. W. et al., 2006. Prevalence of colonisation with group B Streptococci in pregnant women of a multi-ethnic population in The Netherlands. *Eur J Obstet Gynecol Reprod Biol,* 124(2), pp. 178-83.

Valkenburg-van den Berg, A. W., Sprij, A. J., Dekker, F. W., et al., 2009. Association between colonization with Group B Streptococcus and preterm delivery: a systematic review. *Acta Obst Gyn Scand,* 88(9), pp. 958-967.

van der Ham, D. P., van der Heyden, J. L., Opmeer, B. C., et al., 2012a. Management of late-preterm premature rupture of membranes: the PPROMEXIL-2 trial. *AJOG,* 207(276), p. e1–10.

van der Ham, D. P., Vijgen, S. M. Nijhuis, J. G., et al., 2012b. Induction of labor versus expectant management in women with preterm prelabor rupture of membranes between 34 and 37 weeks: a randomized controlled trial. *PLoS Med*, 9(e1001208).

Vergnano, S., Embleton, N., Collinson, A., et al., 2010. Missed opportunities for preventing group B streptococcus infection. *Arch Dis Childhood: Fet Neonat Ed*, 95(1), pp. F72-F73.

Vergnano, S., Menson, E., Kennea, N. & Embleton, N., 2011. Neonatal infections in England: the NeonIN surveillance network. *Arch Dis Child Fetal Neonatal Ed*. 96(1), pp. F9-F14.

Wang, L. Y., Chen, C. T., Liu, W. H., et al., 2007. Recurrent neonatal group B streptococcal disease associated with infected breast milk. *Clin Pediatrics*, 46(6), pp. 547-549.

Watts, G., 2014. UK declares war on antimicrobial resistance. *The Lancet*, 384(391).

Whitney, C., Daly, S., Limpongsanurak, S., et al., 2004. The International Infections in Pregnancy Study: group B streptococcal colonization in pregnant women. *J Mat-Fetal Neonat Med*, 15(4), pp. 267-274.

Wickham, S., 2009. Screening and the consequences of knowledge. *Birthspirit Midwifery Journal*, Volume 2, pp. 9-12.

Wickham, S., 2014. *Inducing Labour: making informed decisions*. Surbiton: AIMS.

Yagupsky, P., Menegus, M. A. & Powell, K. R., 1991. The changing spectrum of group B streptococcal disease in infants: an eleven-year experience in a tertiary care hospital. *Ped Infect Dis J*, Volume 10, pp. 801-8.

Yancey, M. K. et al., 1996. The accuracy of late antenatal screening cultures in predicting genital group B streptococcal colonization at delivery. *O&G*, 88(5), pp. 811-5.

Zanetti-Dällenbach, R., Lapaire, O., Holzgreve, W. & Hösli, I., 2007. Neonatal Colonization-Rate with Group B Streptococcus is Lower in Neonates Born Underwater than after Conventional Vaginal Delivery. *Geburtshilfe Frauenheilkd*, 67(10), pp. 1114-1119.

Zanetti-Dällenbach, R. et al., 2006. Water birth: is the water an additional reservoir for group B streptococcus? *Arch Gynecol Obstet*, 273(4), pp. 236-8.

Zilberman, D., Williams, S. F., Kurian R., et al., 2014. Does genital tract GBS colonization affect the latency period in patients with preterm premature rupture of membranes not in labor prior to 34 weeks? *J Mat-Fet Neonat Med*, 27(4), pp. 338-341.

Resources

AIMS is a voluntary organisation which provides independent support and information about maternity choices. AIMS has a confidential helpline Tel: 0300 365 0663 or helpline@aims.org.uk staffed by dedicated volunteers. AIMS actively supports parents and healthcare professionals who recognise that, for the majority of women, birth is a normal rather than a medical event. www.aims.org.uk

Birthrights is a UK organisation dedicated to improving women's experience of pregnancy and childbirth by promoting respect for human rights. www.birthrights.org.uk

Group B Strep Support is a charity which provides information about GBS for women in the UK, although their information is geared towards recommending screening and antibiotics. They campaign for culture-based screening in the UK and keep an up-to-date list of laboratories which offer private testing in the UK at gbss.org.uk/what-is-gbs/testing-for-gbs/ecm-test-where-how/

www.sarawickham.com contains hundreds of free articles and blog posts for anyone seeking information about birth and midwifery. As GBS is a key interest of Sara's, there are a number of GBS-related blog posts and articles on the website (including several of those in the reference list) and it is worth searching this website as Sara writes a twice-weekly blog which often includes updates on recent research.

Dr Sara Wickham PhD, RM, MA, PGCert, BA(Hons) is a midwife, educator, writer and researcher who works independently, dividing her working time between speaking, writing, blogging, facilitating workshops, creating resources for midwives, birth workers and women and undertaking a wide variety of consultancy and advisory activities. Sara's career has been varied and includes twenty years of experience as a midwife, lecturer and researcher. She is the author/editor of thirteen books, has lectured in more than twenty countries, edited two midwifery journals and provides consultancy services for midwifery and health-related organisations around the world. Her website can be found at www.sarawickham.com

Index

Was the information in this book helpful to you? Please let us know your views of this book. Particularly, if you think there is information that could be included, or amended. Send your views to: feedback@aims.org.uk

Other publications published or sold by AIMS can be ordered from the AIMS website – www.aims.org.uk/?pubs.htm

- Am I Allowed?

- Birth After Caesarean

- Birthing Your Baby: The Second Stage

- Birthing Your Placenta: The Third Stage

- Breech Birth - What are my options?

- Inducing Labour - Making Informed Decisions

- Safety in Childbirth

- Making a Complaint about Maternity Care

- Ultrasound? Unsound

- Vitamin K and the Newborn

- What's Right for Me? - Making decisions in pregnancy and birth

- Caesarean Birth - Your Questions Answered

We are pleased to offer some of these books on Kindle, so you can read them on Kindle readers, tablets, smart phones, PCs and other devices order from www.aims.org.uk/?aboutKindle.htm

AiMS

There for your mother
Here for you
Help us to be there for your daughters

www.aims.org.uk

Twitter – @AIMS_online

Facebook – www.facebook.com/AIMSUK

Helpline
helpline@aims.org.uk
0300 365 0663